Cochlear Implantation in Adults

Wiebke Rötz • Bodo Bertram

Cochlear Implantation in Adults

Care and Rehabilitation in Speech and Language Therapy

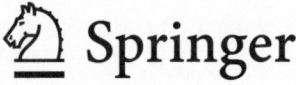 Springer

Wiebke Rötz
Bad Salzuflen, Germany

Bodo Bertram
Berlin, Germany

ISBN 978-3-662-72229-9   ISBN 978-3-662-72230-5   (eBook)
https://doi.org/10.1007/978-3-662-72230-5

This book is a translation of the original German edition "Cochlea Implantat bei Erwachsenen" by Wiebke Rötz and Bodo Bertram, published by Springer-Verlag GmbH, DE in 2022. The translation was done with the help of an artificial intelligence machine translation tool. A subsequent human revision was done primarily in terms of content, so that the book will read stylistically differently from a conventional translation. Springer Nature works continuously to further the development of tools for the production of books and on the related technologies to support the authors.

Translation from the German language edition: "Cochlea Implantat bei Erwachsenen" by Wiebke Rötz and Bodo Bertram, © Der/die Herausgeber bzw. der/die Autor(en), exklusiv lizenziert an Springer-Verlag GmbH, DE, ein Teil von Springer Nature 2022. Published by Springer Berlin Heidelberg. All Rights Reserved.

© The Editor(s) (if applicable) and The Author(s), under exclusive license to Springer-Verlag GmbH, DE, part of Springer Nature 2025

This work is subject to copyright. All rights are solely and exclusively licensed by the Publisher, whether the whole or part of the material is concerned, specifically the rights of translation, reprinting, reuse of illustrations, recitation, broadcasting, reproduction on microfilms or in any other physical way, and transmission or information storage and retrieval, electronic adaptation, computer software, or by similar or dissimilar methodology now known or hereafter developed.

The use of general descriptive names, registered names, trademarks, service marks, etc. in this publication does not imply, even in the absence of a specific statement, that such names are exempt from the relevant protective laws and regulations and therefore free for general use.

The publisher, the authors and the editors are safe to assume that the advice and information in this book are believed to be true and accurate at the date of publication. Neither the publisher nor the authors or the editors give a warranty, expressed or implied, with respect to the material contained herein or for any errors or omissions that may have been made. The publisher remains neutral with regard to jurisdictional claims in published maps and institutional affiliations.

This Springer imprint is published by the registered company Springer-Verlag GmbH, DE, part of Springer Nature.
The registered company address is: Heidelberger Platz 3, 14197 Berlin, Germany

If disposing of this product, please recycle the paper.

Foreword

Dear ladies and gentlemen, dear readers,

I am very pleased that with this book a consideration of the hearing-speech therapeutic rehabilitation after cochlear implantation is now available for a broad, multi-professional readership.

In addition to the medical-surgical view on the topic complex and the technical, audiological, electrophysiological perception of the "Cochlear Implantation," the hearing-speech therapeutic contribution is the third mainstay.

The interprofessional exchange of these groups is the basis for high-quality care, follow-up, and accompaniment after a cochlear implantation.

This book is aimed at a broad, multi-professional readership and thus creates a broad understanding for the hearing-speech therapeutic approach.

This approach has developed, structured, and selected in the last decades of care with cochlear implants.

The author team picks up this development in an excellent way. On the one hand, it combines invaluable experience due to decades of care for cochlear implant patients with the development of initial rehabilitative concepts from the early days of CI care, and on the other hand, experiences with speech therapeutic care under telemedical conditions and the development of therapeutic AI-based app concepts.

Warm greetings and enjoy reading!

Managing Senior Physician of the Clinic for Ear, Nose, Otorhinolaryngology of the University Hospital Bielefeld Campus Mitte, Medical Faculty OWL Bielefeld, Germany

P. D. Dr. med. I. Todt

Preface

The Cochlear Implant (CI) is the first fully functioning electronic sensory prosthesis that takes over the function of the defective inner ear. So far, over 500,000 patients worldwide have been able to benefit from this impressive technology. However, in daily work with adult CI patients and in exchange with other therapists, it becomes clear that the development of suitable therapeutic concepts for adults' lags behind the offer for CI-supplied children in many respects.

Already in the 1990s, Dr. Bodo Bertram, as educational director at the Cochlear Implant Centre (CIC) "Wilhelm Hirte" in Hanover (Germany), established a structured care for children with CI, thus making a tremendous contribution to the care of hearing-impaired children after cochlear implantation. The therapy center was at this time the only one of its kind worldwide and became a model for therapy centers all over the world in the following years.

If a child gains access to spoken language for the first time through a CI, however, a different form of therapy is needed than with CI care in adulthood, when the already learned verbal spoken language must be newly recognized and assigned with the CI. For those affected, the chance to regain long-missed hearing and understanding, as well as to regain communication skills that enable improved social interaction, is also essential.

The accompaniment of patients in the decision-making process and in the therapy process therefore includes much more than just exercise treatment. Preoperative clarification on all questions of CI care, its possibilities, and detailed information on the limits and risks of this intervention and on the goals of evidence-based postoperative rehabilitation are just some of the topics. Concrete guidance on how to carry out such therapy and accompany patients with hearing loss adequately is discussed in different sources, but it is missing in the sense of a therapy guideline for therapists.

This gap is to be filled by the book for all therapists in speech and hearing therapy: orientation and basic knowledge for all steps of CI care and guidance for therapy. It offers theoretical knowledge and practical accompaniment of therapy using the example of care in Germany and is supplemented by scientific findings with experiences from many years of practical work. It was also important to us to highlight the interdisciplinary exchange between surgery, audiology, and therapy, which significantly improves hearing success with the CI.

For the future, and especially in the context of the increasing academization of therapeutic professions in Germany, we wish for a progressive scientific examination of the aspects of speech and hearing therapy. Only in this way can therapy for people with a CI be designed individually, resource-saving and at the same time evidence-based.

Bad Salzuflen, Germany   Wiebke Rötz
Berlin, Germany   Bodo Bertram

Acknowledgments

I would like to express my heartfelt thanks to W. Rötz, who asked me to contribute to this book on the history of cochlear implants and on aspects of the collaboration between doctors, therapists, and future as well as already CI-supplied adult patients. I was very happy to comply with her request.

Working with her was very pleasant, cooperative, and characterized by a constant exchange of arguments. Rötz has driven the joint project forward with compelling competence and impressive diligence.

I would also like to express my sincere thanks to PD Dr. Todt for his willingness to review my contributions from a medical perspective.

I wish the book much success. It contains a valuable and extensive treasure of methodological approaches for the postoperative therapeutic accompaniment of CI-supplied adult patients. In combination with the indispensable therapeutic creativity of each therapist, it provides unique assistance.

Dr. rer. biol. hum. Bodo Bertram

The very different times at which Dr. B. Bertram and I have experienced the development of CI care in Germany and the various tasks in our work with CI-supplied people over the years make the content of the book a special collection of knowledge and experience. For the close exchange, the impulses brought in, and the valuable contributions in the book, I would like to express my sincere thanks to Dr. Bertram.

I would also like to express special thanks to my colleague PD Dr. I. Todt, who was always supportive, motivating, and above all stood by with his ENT medical expertise, as well as my audiological colleague and friend Theda Eichler for her professional assessment and support in the creation process of the book.

Last but not least, my husband, my family, and friends were a great help in implementing the book idea through their tireless proofreading and encouragement during the work-intensive months, for which I am very grateful.

Wiebke Rötz

Contents

1 Basics of the Cochlear Implant (CI) 1
  1.1 Historical Development of the CI 1
  1.2 Causes of CI-Relevant Hearing Disorders 6
  1.3 Structure and Functioning of the CI 7
  1.4 CI Manufacturers 10
  1.5 Implants 11
  1.6 Sound Processors 14
  1.7 Opportunities in the Fitting of Sound Processors 18
  Literature 21

2 Needs of Patients in the Care Process 25
  2.1 Importance of Hearing Ability and Hearing Loss 25
  2.2 CI Indication: Changes from 1984 to 2020 29
  2.3 CI as a Chance for a New Beginning 33
  2.4 Right to Comprehensive Preoperative Information 36
  Literature 39

3 Variants of Therapy 41
  3.1 Concept Clarification 41
  3.2 Audio Therapy 42
  3.3 Auditory Training 44
  3.4 Connectivity and Accessories 52
  Literature 60

4 Preparation of the Therapy 63
  4.1 Coordination Between Surgery, Audiology, and Therapy 63
  4.2 Anamnesis Based on the International Classification
       of Functioning, Disability and Health (ICF) 65
  4.3 Diagnostics and Findings 69
  4.4 Goals Based on the ICF 72
  Literature 74

5	**Structure and Contents of Therapy**	77
	5.1 Exercise Areas and Their Implementation	78
	5.2 Feedback to the Patient	99
	5.3 Feedback to the Audiology Department	109
	Literature	113
6	**Exercise Instructions and Materials for Auditory Training**	115
	6.1 Exercises of Linguistic Exercise Areas	115
	6.2 Exercises for Nonlinguistic Exercise Areas	130

Glossary ... 137

Index ... 139

Abbreviations

ABI	Auditory Brainstem Implant
ACIR	Working Group for Cochlear Implant Rehabilitation
ADANO	Working Group of German Audiologists, Neurootologists and Otologists
AHL	Asymmetric Hearing Loss
BDH	Professional Association of German Educators of the Hearing Impaired
CIC	Cochlear Implant Centre Hannover
C-Level	Comfort Level
CROS	Contralateral Routing of Signals
dbl e.V.	German Federal Association for Speech and Language Therapy (registered association)
DCIG	German Cochlear Implant Society (registered association)
DGA	German Society for Audiology
DGNR	German Society for Neuroradiology
DGPP	German Society for Phoniatrics and Pediatric Audiology (registered association)
DSB	German Association for the Hearing Impaired (registered association)
EAS	Electroacoustic Stimulation
E-BERA	"Brainstem Evoked Response Audiometry" through direct electrical stimulation of the auditory nerve
EUHA	European Union of Hearing Aid Professionals (registered association)
HdO-Processor	Behind-the-Ear Processor
ICF	International Classification of Functioning, Disability and Health
SSD	Single-Sided-Deafness
TICI	Totally Implantable Cochlear Implant
T-Level	Threshold Level
WHO	World Health Organization

Basics of the Cochlear Implant (CI)

1.1 Historical Development of the CI

Bodo Bertram

The following explanations on the history of the CI can only provide a cursory insight into the fascinating development of the CI over the past decades within the scope of this book.

International research has laid the foundation for the successful symptomatic treatment of existing inner ear deafness. Affected individuals are now able to hear spoken language again and thus regain good speech comprehension.

For deaf-born children, the CI enables for the first time in the history of deaf education and upbringing, with excellent therapeutic guidance from parents and professionals, the hearing-supported acquisition of a spoken language competence at a high level, provided all prerequisites for this are given. The CI—an impressive and revolutionary invention.

> Making deaf people hear has always been a dream of committed scientists and otologists.

The Italian physicist Alessandro Volta (1745–1827) already conducted a self-experiment. He inserted two wires connected to a battery into the outer ear canals to find out whether electrical hearing was possible. However, Volta wasn't deaf, but hearing (1.Lehnhardt 1998).

The realization by Wever and Bray (1936) that bioelectric currents are involved in the transmission of acoustic information from the sensory organ to the auditory nerve—so-called microphone potentials—led to the hope: "If it were possible to reproduce the pattern of spikes triggered by them in the auditory nerve, then a sensation of hearing could also be achieved beyond the dead inner ear" (Lehnhardt 1998 ibid.). However, this raised the question of how to achieve an understanding of speech.

© The Author(s), under exclusive license to Springer-Verlag GmbH, DE, part of Springer Nature 2025
W. Rötz, B. Bertram, *Cochlear Implantation in Adults*,
https://doi.org/10.1007/978-3-662-72230-5_1

The Frenchmen André Djourno (physicist) and Charles Eyriès (otologist) were able to prove as early as 1957 that "sensations of hearing could be triggered by electrical stimulation of the auditory nerve" (Battmer 2009). Djourno had demonstrated in animal experiments that even after countless electrical excitations of the auditory nerve, the nerve substance remained unchanged. His hope was that the auditory nerve of the deaf could be directly stimulated with such potentials. The prerequisite for this was necessarily functioning auditory nerve fibers. On February 25, 1957, the first patient was provided with this developed CI. Compared to today, the results were still very modest. "Sensations of hearing were limited to cricket chirping, crunching or whistling" (Lehnhardt 1998 loc. cit., p. 2 ff.). The "Hamburger Morgenpost" reported on this sensational success in its edition of August 17th in 1957 under the title: "Radio in the Head" (Hamburger Morgenpost 1957).

These research results were an impetus for further research worldwide. The goal was to achieve a soon clinical application of future CI.

It is worth highlighting a wrongly little noticed pioneering achievement of two German researchers for CI research—the otologist Frank Zöllner and the sensory physiologist Wolf-Dieter Keidel. As early as 1963, they had inserted an electrode through the round window into the cochlea in two patients with unilateral Menière's disease during a vestibular labyrinthectomy under local anesthesia. Thus, the patients were able to describe their hearing impressions in detail. These findings led to proposals by Zöllner and Keidel for the implementation of a future speech-conveying implant. They are to be recognized as a significant pioneering achievement for CI development.

Proposals for the implementation of a speech-conveying implant by Zöllner and Keidel

1. "Transcutaneous transmission
2. Platinum electrodes of 0.35 mm diameter
3. Placed intracochlearly
4. Distributed over the frequency range of preferably 300–3000 Hz
5. In a number of 20 (100)
6. Emphasis on location coding" Lehnhardt 1998 (loc. cit., p. 4 f.)

In addition, a device (sound processor) was needed that converts the received spoken language into electrical patterns.

1.1 Historical Development of the CI

Today's implants show a very impressive correspondence with the proposals of these two researchers.

William House and Jack Urban in Los Angeles implanted the first electrodes in 1961, followed by a single-channel implant at the House Ear Institute in 1972. Their research contributed significantly to the fact that "the CI was introduced from research into clinical routine and thus directly benefited the deaf (House and Urban 1973)" (Battmer 2009, 1).

Additional groups such as

- Simmons, Stanford University, 1966
- Chouard, Paris, 1973
- Graeme Clark in Melbourne, 1979
- Burian Hochmair-Desoyer and Hochmair in Vienna
- Banfai in Düren, 1975
- Dillier and Spielmann, Zurich, 1976
- Fraysse in Toulouse
- Hrubý and Tichý in Prague

researched the implementation of a clinically applicable CI (Lehnhardt 1998 a.a.O. pp. 4–6 f.).

During this phase, further significant questions arose for the CI research, which were discussed very controversially within the international research groups:

- Single-channel or multichannel
- Placement of the electrode array: extracochlear or intracochlear
- Percutaneous or transcutaneous transmission

All implants used today are multichannel, intracochlear with positioning of the electrode array in the scala tympani. A special surgical procedure is indicated when malformations or an obliteration or ossification of the cochlea are present.

The achievements of the scientists contributed to the fact that today's implants convey such a high degree of speech understanding. But also, the patients who have been provided with them have made a significant contribution to these successes. They have confidently turned to the new technology and provided the scientists with crucial clues about hearing and understanding speech with the CI. This knowledge, in turn, led to the constant further development of increasingly efficient speech coding strategies.

1.1.1 Beginning and Course of the Clinical Application of the CI

In August 1978, Clark implanted the world's first multichannel 16-electrode cochlear encompassing (CI) system. The transmission was transcutaneous, i.e., through the intact skin using a portable sound processor (Clark et al. 1978). In 1980, the scientific cooperation between the University of Melbourne and Nucleus Ltd.,

Sydney, began with the goal of developing the first transcutaneous, intracochlear, multichannel implant system.

In 1978, P. Banfai in Düren–Birkenhof was the first in Germany to implant a CI developed by him in collaboration with Hortmann and Kubik. The signal transmission was percutaneous, i.e., via a plug through the skin. This was associated with the risk of future and dangerous infections. The goal of the extracochlear supply was to protect the highly sensitive cochlear nerve from damage. The hoped-for successes regarding speech understanding, however, did not materialize (Schnecke 2018). The poor image of the implant contributed significantly to the massive resentments in the deaf community against the CI providers of deaf toddlers to this day.

In 1984, E. Lehnhardt decided together with R-D. Battmer for the Australian implant Nucleus. Battmer gave the decisive impetus for this. The recommendations presented by Keidel and Zöllner for the development of future cochlear implants, which were applied in this system, among other things, were decisive for this decision. In this regard, together with R. Laszig, the CI supply and comprehensive research in Hannover were driven forward.

Due to the impressive postoperative successes in Hannover regarding speech comprehension with the CI, other German clinics subsequently decided to provide CI care.

At that time, additional implants were available as alternatives, such as a French one from Chouard, the already mentioned Düren CI from Banfai and Hortmann, the Vienna CI from Burian and Hochmair, as well as the Zurich CI from Dillier/Spillmann, and finally the House-Institute-CI. The multichannel implants were intracochlear models. An exception was the extracochlear multichannel system originally manufactured by the Hortmann company, which Banfai used in a modified form (Laubert 1986).

For clinical application, it was crucial that the implants had to prove effective and safe, and that for many years. A significant finding was that a defective implant could usually be explanted without major complications. This knowledge was also the decisive prerequisite also for the CI supply for children.

In 1988, Lehnhardt operated on a deaf-born toddler for the first time at the ENT-Clinic of the Medical University of Hannover with the Nucleus Mini System 22, as this model was suitable for the child's skull due to its size. The CI supply for children was associated with the demand to establish a postoperative concept for the hearing-aided hearing and speech development of deaf-born and deafened children. With the Cochlear Implant Centrum Hannover (CIC), initiated by Lehnhardt, a facility was available for the first time worldwide in 1990 that implemented this claim (Bertram 1991, 1992).

A significant milestone was also the development of brainstem implants, which enabled patients with central hearing disorders (bilaterally nonfunctional auditory nerves) to experience hearing sensations and understand speech through electrical stimulation at the still functional auditory nerve nucleus. R. Laszig is credited with being the first surgeon in Europe to have implanted a brainstem implant in 1993 (Laszig 1993).

1.1 Historical Development of the CI

In addition to the reliability of the CI systems, it was necessary to find ways to uniformly define failures of implants or their faulty operation (the implant can no longer fulfill its specified functions) to clearly distinguish them from possible medical causes. For this purpose, an international expert group was formed, which was to develop criteria for the definition of the failure of an implant (Battmer 2009 a.a.O., S. 3-4 f.). Both technical and medical causes were taken into account.

Among other things, additional safety checks can be used: "Ultimately, the objective methods of CI monitoring are available to exclude postoperative complications or to determine the causes of rehabilitation disorders" (Basta 2009). Procedures such as the E-BERA and the stapedius reflex measurement also contribute to making statements about the function of the further auditory pathways from a medical point of view (Battmer 2009, ibid.).

The success of postoperative (Re-)Habilitation is, among many other factors, significantly influenced by the quality of the developed sound processor. This situation applies to both adult patients and CI-supplied children.

Finally, Ernst and Todt (2009) demand as the goal of every CI surgeon "[...] to insert the implant and especially the electrode as atraumatically and gently as possible during the operative procedure, in order to minimize the burden on the patient while maintaining high quality of care." They refer to the "soft-surgery-technique" (Lehnhardt 1993).

1.1.2 Further Developments in CI Supply

The last three decades have been characterized by a multitude of developments. This included the increasing miniaturization of implants, the associated use of new electrode arrays, as well as the miniaturization of sound processors, preprocessing, and the development of more efficient speech coding strategies. New surgical procedures minimize operation risks and the insertion trauma of the cochlear implant; the stresses on patients caused by the surgical intervention are reduced.

Another crucial advancement was the bilateral CI supply for the severely hearing-impaired. It is now a standard supply, which has proven to provide better speech understanding in noise, as well as better directional hearing (Müller et al. 2000; Laszig et al. 2004). Bilaterally supplied patients report "a significant relief of listening in the sense of a lesser necessary hearing effort. This improves the ability to communicate verbally in the mostly noisy hearing situations of everyday life" (Müller-Deile and Laszig 2009).

Electro-acoustic stimulation (EAS) (v. Ilberg 1999) is a significant milestone in the treatment of patients with residual hearing in the low-frequency range and allows for the use of hybrid implants to preserve residual hearing.

The cochlear implant for single-sided deafness (SSD; Van de Heyning et al. 2008; Arndt et al. 2011); the implantation of the totally implantable cochlear implant (TICI; Robert et al. 2008), which is not yet routine clinical practice and requires further research (Müller 2021); and the molecular biology-based inner ear therapy, drug-releasing electrodes (MED-EL 2021), to avoid inflammation and achieve unhindered transmission of the hearing signal between electrode and auditory nerve, are further highlights of this rapid development.

1.1.3 Current Developments in CI Research

New visions and research enable continuous development:

"Hearing with light" (Animal experiments understand 2021)—a promising technique that aims for a significant improvement of hearing with the CI, due to a high number of electrodes on the electrode array is assumed to have about 60–100 electrodes.

The use of telemetry allows for intraoperative function control of the implants. CI remote fitting saves the patients from long trips to the clinic. The use of surgical robots, the use of nanotechnology for self-forming electrodes with higher conductivity, the preoperative measurement of the cochlea, the use of new navigation techniques for malformations of the cochlea, rotation tomography or 3D volume CT, and the increasing digitization of collected patient data and telemedicine are further focuses in the constantly developing CI supply.

In 1996, the author founded the Working Group Cochlear Implant (Re-)Habilitation (ACIR) in Hanover, which now includes 20 therapy centers that provide both inpatient and outpatient services for postoperative treatment of CI-supplied patients at a high level. The employees of these centers dedicate themselves with great commitment and empathy to this task.

1.2 Causes of CI-Relevant Hearing Disorders

Wiebke Rötz

The indication for CI supply exists when the audiological criteria and the anatomical and pathophysiological conditions are met. These are almost exclusively cochlear severe hearing impairments of great extent (Battmer 2009). This means that verbal understanding with hearing aids is no longer possible, and the stimulability of the auditory nerve is present. Retrocochlear structures such as the auditory nerve and the central components of the hearing process must be intact (Diller 1997). Various cochlear causes can influence the later success with the CI (Sect. 2.2). The following discusses common causes that can influence rehabilitation.

The most common causes are unclear causes, genetic diseases, acute hearing loss, and traumas in the sense of temporal bone fractures or acoustic events.

There is a correlation between the duration of deafness and the achieved speech audiometric result in relation to the time of rehabilitation duration (Leung et al. 2005). This means that a short duration of deafness usually requires a short rehabilitation to achieve a good to very good result with the CI.

For specific patient groups, the conditions for care with a CI must be particularly considered.

As a result of Menière's disease (symptom triad: hearing loss, vertigo, tinnitus), hearing ability can be significantly impaired. Due to the often-impaired balance function, the reduction in quality of life starting from the vertigo complaints is usually much greater than due to the severe hearing loss (Zeh 2011). In addition to the specific form of surgical care for this patient group, the lack of focus on hearing-speech training often slows down the rehabilitation process after successful implantation.

As a result of meningitis or labyrinthitis, not only can deafness occur, but also obliterations and ossifications of the cochlea. This requires close imaging control (CT, MRI) and possibly timely implantation (Aschendorff et al. 2005, 2009). Otherwise, a complete insertion of the electrode array could be difficult, and due to a partial insertion, the result with the CI could be impaired.

In the case of benign neoplasms within the cochlea (e.g., intralabyrinthine schwannomas), both the removal of the schwannomas and successful care with a CI can be carried out. In the case of benign neoplasms outside the cochlea (e.g., vestibular schwannomas), care may be indicated in individual cases if the auditory nerve is functional. Here, it is necessary to coordinate the therapeutic approaches regarding surgery, radiation, or watchful waiting, as well as the audiological rehabilitation (Ernst and Todt 2009; Wick et al. 2020).

In general, as a result of regular middle ear operations (cholesteatoma operations, tympanoplasties, etc.), there is the possibility of damaging the hearing. The resulting indication for subsequent CI care must be clarified in the individual case.

1.3 Structure and Functioning of the CI

Wiebke Rötz

The CI system consists of an implant and a sound processor. Only when there is contact between both components via the transmitter and receiver coil, information is transferred from the sound processor to the implant, so that a hearing impression can be created.

1.3.1 The External Part

A sound processor (Fig. 1.1) always includes an energy-supplying unit, microphones, the actual sound processor, and a transmitter coil with a magnet. Depending on the type of sound processor, there is also a coil cable, which connects the sound processor with the transmitter coil, and an ear hook, which allows the sound processor to sit on the ear.

Fig. 1.1 Naída CI M Sound processor. (Courtesy of Advanced Bionics. All rights reserved)

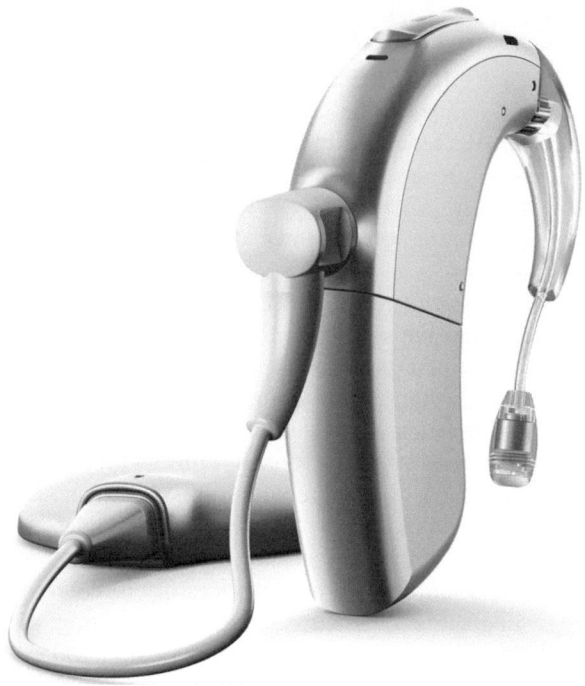

All sound processors or transmitter coils can be removed at any time, as the transmitter coil only holds on the head by a magnet on the closed skin. The information and energy transfer thus takes place transcutaneously.

Power Supply
Depending on the specific model, the sound processors are powered by either disposable or rechargeable batteries. This provides the power supply for both the sound processor and the implant.

Microphones
All current sound processors have at least two microphones, which pick up sound from the outside. A number of at least two microphones is important to form directional characteristics. These are necessary to improve directional hearing and hearing and understanding in noise.

Sound Processor
The term sound processor or processor is generally used. Sometimes, the term speech processor is also found in the literature.

The captured sound is processed according to the programmed settings, converted into electrical impulses, and forwarded to the transmitter coil.

1.3 Structure and Functioning of the CI

Transmitter Coil with Magnet

The transmitter coil of the behind-the-ear processors (BTE processors) or the single-unit processors is attached to the implant using a magnet. The transmitter coil sends the previously received information and the required energy inductively to the implant.

Inductive Transmission

In the case of the CI, the inductive transmission takes place via the two very closely located coils: the transmitter and the receiver coil. Energy and information are transferred to the receiver coil via an electromagnetic field. As soon as the coils move away from each other, the contact is interrupted. The correct positioning of the transmitter coil is therefore essential for reliable transmission (Rahne 2021; Trieu et al. 2009; Kramme 2011; Lenarz 2017).

1.3.2 The Implantable Part

An implant (Fig. 1.2) always consists of a receiver coil, a magnet, a stimulator, an electrode array, and the electrodes.

Receiver Coil with Magnet

The receiver coil receives the signal, which is transmitted by the transmitter coil of the sound processor. The magnet holds the external part on the head.

Stimulator

In the stimulator, the signal received from the sound processor is decoded and converted into electrical impulses. In the literature, this is also referred to as the electronics or the receiver.

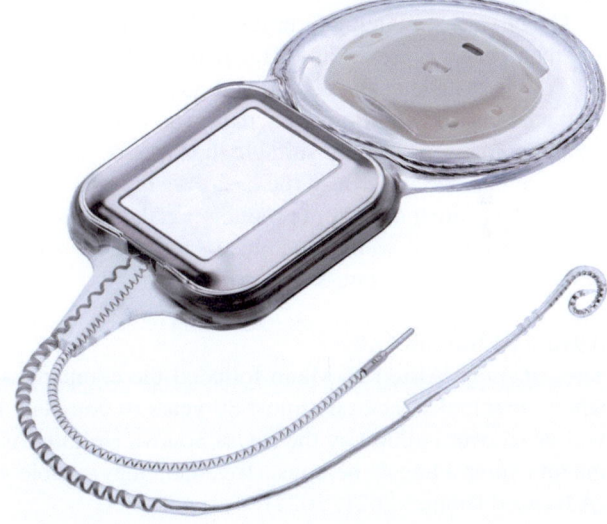

Fig. 1.2 Cochlear™ Nucleus® Profile Plus with Contour Advance® electrode (CI612). (Courtesy of Cochlear. © Cochlear Limited 2022. All rights reserved)

Electrode Array
The electrode contacts are mounted on the electrode array. The section at the tip of the electrode array is inserted into the cochlea during surgery and is often synonymously referred to as the electrode. The electrical impulses are passed on to the electrode contacts in the cochlea via the electrode array.

Electrodes
Depending on the manufacturer, an implant has 12–22 electrodes, which are inserted into the cochlea and represent the interface to the auditory nerve endings. In addition, each implant has electrodes that divert the current supplied (cf. Aschendorff et al. 2009; Adunka and Kiefer 2005; Büchner and Gärtner 2017; Lenarz 2017; Müller-Deile 2009).

1.4 CI Manufacturers

Wiebke Rötz

At the present time, patients in Germany are supplied with CI from the companies Advanced Bionics, Cochlear®, and MED-EL. Oticon Medical was also among the common manufacturers, but was recently taken over by Cochlear®. As patients are still being supplied with Oticon Medical, this manufacturer will also be discussed in the following. All manufacturers regularly develop new implants and sound processors every few years.

Internationally, there is another CI manufacturer, which is headquartered in the People's Republic of China. This is the company Nurotron®, which should only be mentioned for the sake of completeness (Medical EXPO 2024). Since there is no experience with this manufacturer in Germany, it will not be discussed further in the following chapters.

The choice of manufacturer depends on the individual conditions of the patient and their personal preference. The treating ENT doctor, preferably the surgeon himself, discusses and evaluates the individual conditions with the patient. In this context, anatomical conditions may make the implantation of a certain implant from a manufacturer appear more suitable than others. Ultimately, a decision must always be recommended in favor of the best possible hearing success. This must always be seen in the context of current products and developments. Due to the high variability of new products as well as technical and surgical solutions, the clinic must always have several manufacturers at hand.

Advanced Bionics (AB)
The American Alfred E. Mann founded the company Advanced Bionics in 1993, which now looks back on almost 30 years of company history. Most recently, AB was taken over in 2009 by the Swiss Sonova Holding AG, to which the hearing aid manufacturer Phonak belongs. Together, they enable bimodal hearing solutions (Advanced Bionics 2021, 2022).

Cochlear®
Cochlear® is an Australian company and originated from the research work of Graeme Clark, who implanted the first multichannel CI in 1978. The company Cochlear® was formed in 1981 from the collaboration of the Nucleus Group with the Australian government. Since 2017, Cochlear® and the hearing aid manufacturer GN Resound have been offering bimodal hearing solutions (ReSound 2022; Cochlear 2021).

MED-EL
The Austrian company MED-EL was founded in 1990 by Ingeborg and Erwin Hochmair and has its headquarters in Innsbruck. However, the foundation was preceded by many years of research since 1975. In Germany, the subsidiary MED-EL Elektromedizinische Geräte Deutschland operates and is the contact for all concerns of patients and professional staff (MED-EL 2022b, c, d, e).

Oticon Medical (OM)
The Danish hearing aid manufacturer Oticon was founded in 1904 by Hans Demant and taken over in 1910 by his son William Demant, who commercialized the products and under whose leadership the constant development of new hearing aids was driven forward. In 2008, Oticon Medical was founded by the Demant Group, whose first product was a bone-anchored hearing device. In 2013, the French manufacturer Neurelec was taken over, thereby additionally expanding the area of was added to the portfolio. The acquired technology was then adapted to Oticon standards, and bimodal hearing solutions were created. Finally, it was announced that Cochlear® would take over Oticon Medical in the summer of 2022 (Demant 2022; Oticon Medical 2015, 2018).

▶ **Tip** All CI companies have a customer service that can be used by patients as well as by professionals. The respective contact details can be found on the manufacturers' homepages.
  www.advancedbionics.com
  www.cochlear.com
  www.medel.com
  www.oticonmedical.com

1.5 Implants

Wiebke Rötz

The implants of all manufacturers have a low failure rate, which can be proven over long-term observation periods. Therefore, reimplantations are comparatively rare. Should a reimplantation occur, a deterioration of the speech audiometric result is not usually expected.

All manufacturers strive to keep the latest generation of sound processors compatible with older generations of implants (backward compatibility). This provision with the latest generation of sound processors is referred to as an "upgrade."

Patients can thus, depending on the date of implantation, have different implant models despite the latest sound processor. There is no influence on the basic approach in speech therapy by the sound processor or the implant.

1.5.1 Properties of Implants

Position of the Electrode Array
The stimulator of the implant is located and fixed on the skull cap. Only the electrode array is inserted into the cochlea. The electrode array is usually introduced into the scala tympani via the round window. In special anatomical cases or with corresponding preexisting conditions, an insertion into the scala vestibuli can also occur or the electrode array can be introduced into the first turn of the cochlea via an additional access route. The electrode is then gently pushed around the modiolus, the central axis of the cochlea, from basal to apical.

Function of the Electrodes Inside the Cochlea
The task of the individual electrode is to electrically stimulate the locally sited spiral ganglia and thus the auditory nerve and thereby bypassing the defective hair cells. Each electrode is assigned a frequency band.

Number of Electrodes
The number of electrodes varies depending on the manufacturer and does not correlate with speech understanding. The terms electrodes and channels are used synonymously when setting the sound processor.

To understand speech, only a small number of electrodes inside the cochlea are needed. For good speech understanding, and in case of electrode defects, the number of electrodes is higher than the minimum required.

Size and Material of the Implant
The thickness of the implants has been significantly reduced over time, with increasing break resistance. The material concepts have been standardized, so that currently only metal housings, embedded in silicone, are used.

Diameter of the Electrode Array
To serve various anatomical and functional conditions, some manufacturers offer implants with different diameters of the electrode arrays. A larger diameter gives the electrode array (possibly with a stylet, wire) more rigidity and can thus better overcome obstacles such as obliterations or ossifications in the cochlea. Electrodes with a smaller diameter are said to be less traumatic and to increase the likelihood of preserving residual hearing.

1.5 Implants

Shape of the Electrode Array

The shape of various electrode arrays is differentiated into preformed and non-preformed. Preformed electrode arrays fit closely to the modiolus. The distance to the spiral ganglia, to which the electrical signal is transmitted, is therefore smaller. Non-preformed electrode arrays fit closely to the lateral wall of the cochlea. Lateral electrode arrays are said to be, just like the electrode arrays with a smaller diameter, less traumatic and to increase the likelihood of preserving residual hearing.

Length of the Electrode Array

The variation in the length of electrode arrays is partly due to their shape. With preformed electrode arrays, which are placed close to the modiolus, the path to the apex is shorter than along the lateral wall to achieve the same insertion depth. That means a 17-mm-long modiolar electrode reaches approximately the same insertion depth as a 24-mm-long lateral electrode.

Furthermore, shorter electrode arrays were designed to preserve still intact hair cells, and thus residual hearing in the low-frequency range, toward the apex of the cochlea. Longer electrodes are said to be able to cover the frequency spectrum of the cochlea better (Fig. 1.3).

MRI Compatibility

In recent years, all manufacturers have used magnets, which can remain in the implant during MRI examination. This allows for pain-free MRI examinations without the risk of magnet dislocation. However, there are still artifacts in MRI imaging (cf. Aschendorff et al. 2009; Ernst and Todt 2009; Battmer 2009; Lenarz 2017). Since the MRI behavior of the implants depends on the magnet of the related implant, the MRI safety of the implant must be clarified *before the MRI examination* (cf. www.advancedbionics.com, www.cochlear.com, www.medel.com, www.oticonmedical.com).

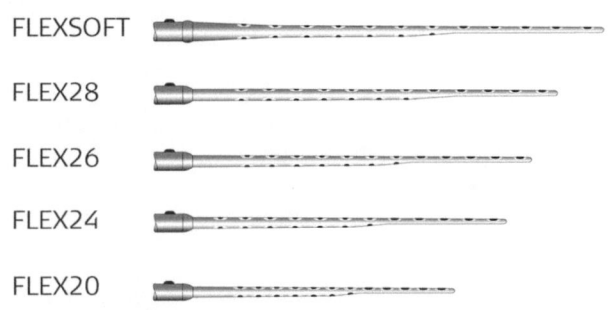

Fig. 1.3 Electrode arrays of the FLEX series from MED-EL for various cochlear conditions. (Courtesy of MED-EL. All rights reserved)

1.6 Sound Processors

Wiebke Rötz

Over the past years, there has been a steady development from once large pocket sound processors (Fig. 1.4) to small, head-worn sound processors. According to the current state, there are two different designs: behind-the-ear processors and the so-called single-unit processors.

The underlying functionality is the same for all sound processors. Which sound processor is best suited for the respective supply depends on the individual conditions of the patient and their personal preferences. The decision for a CI manufacturer is made before the implantation. As part of this selection, the type of sound processor is usually also determined.

1.6.1 Behind-the-Ear Processor

The most common variant is the placement of the sound processor directly behind the ear, hence it is also referred to as a behind-the-ear processor, or in short, BTE processor (Fig. 1.1). In individual cases, a remote placement of the BTE processors is carried out. The BTE processors are equipped with a long coil cable for this purpose and worn on the collar or arm. For adult patients, this may be necessary, for example, when wearing helmets for work-related reasons.

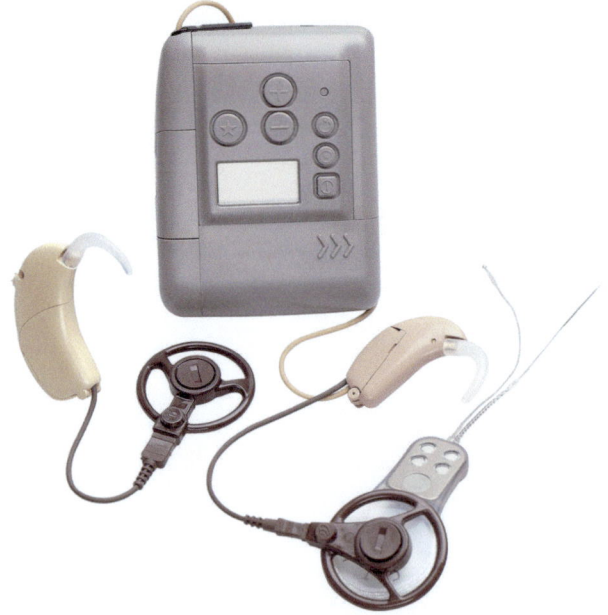

Fig. 1.4 Pocket sound processor with implant. (Courtesy of Cochlear. © Cochlear Limited 2022. All rights reserved)

1.6 Sound Processors

Another special feature is that BTE processors not only stimulate electrically, but also acoustically. These devices form a combination of CI and hearing aid. They are intended for patients who still have residual hearing in the low-frequency range after implantation, which can be amplified with a hearing aid. The BTE processor also has an acoustic unit, which is placed in the ear canal. Depending on the manufacturer, this is referred to as an EAS processor (sound processor for electroacoustic stimulation) or a hybrid sound processor (Fig. 1.5).

▶ With additional acoustic stimulation, patients often need a custom-made earpiece (otoplasty). Some patients wear such earpieces only for better support of the BTE processor on the ear. If the sound processor has an earpiece, it should always be precisely asked what purpose it serves in order to know the exact hearing situation.

Due to the position of the microphones directly on the ear, the sound recording via a BTE processor worn on the head comes closest to natural sound recording. If the implant had to be placed further back, up, or down for medical reasons, BTE processors offer better conditions for picking up sound than a single-unit processor.

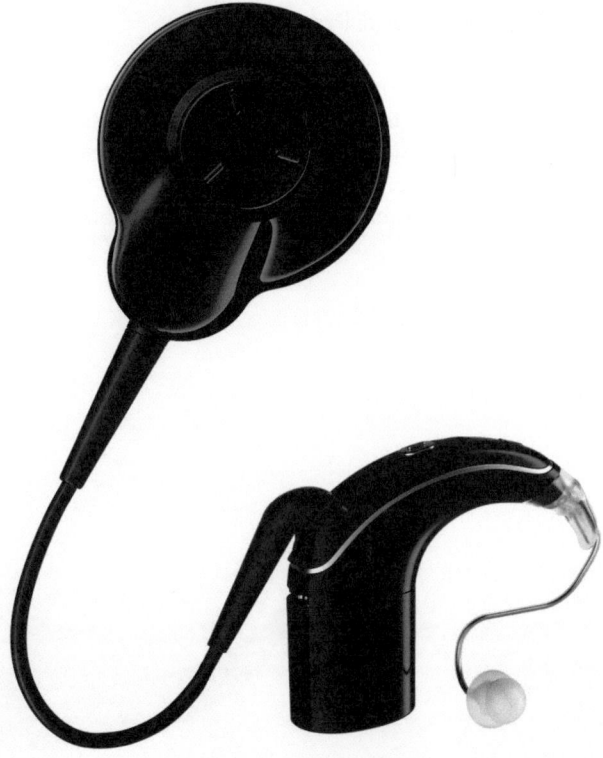

Fig. 1.5 Nucleus® 7 sound processor with Hybrid™ hearing solution for electroacoustic stimulation. (Courtesy of Cochlear. © Cochlear Limited 2022. All rights reserved)

> **Example**
>
> A patient wore a single-unit processor so far back on the head that it was hardly visible from the front. In a quiet environment, the patient could largely understand the spoken word well, but described the speech from behind as clearer. In noise, however, it was hardly possible for the patient to identify spoken words from the front. But when spoken to from behind, she was able to repeat demanding sentences in the noise. ◄

An advantage of BTE processors is the low weight of the transmitter coil compared to the higher weight of the single-unit processor. Especially for patients with thick skin on their head or very firm, protruding hair, the hold of a single-unit processor with the strongest magnet is sometimes not sufficient.

In addition, the transmitter coil of a BTE processor is flatter than a single-unit processor. If a patient often wears a helmet in their free time or is obliged to do so at work, this is more difficult in combination with a single-unit processor.

Since a few factors can only be determined after implantation or during the initial adjustment, a change in the type of sound processor may still be necessary at this point. This can sometimes mean that patients are initially disappointed or question the previous consultation.

1.6.2 Single-Unit Processor

Single-unit processors combine all external components of the CI into one part and are positioned on the implant at a short distance from the ear on the head. This design eliminates the coil cable and the ear hook (Fig. 1.6).

In terms of time, the development of single-unit processors is younger than that of BTE processors, but not all manufacturers offer them. Single-unit processors are

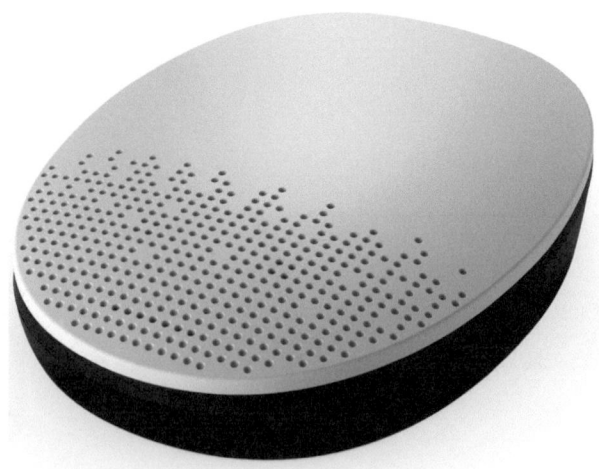

Fig. 1.6 RONDO 3 Sound processor. (Courtesy of MED-EL. All rights reserved)

used when patients do not want to wear the sound processor behind the ear for cosmetic reasons or if placement behind the ear is not possible or only with difficulty.

Electroacoustic stimulation (EAS or Hybrid) is not possible with single-unit processors.

Single-unit processors offer a clear advantage for people with malformations of the outer ear or very closely fitting auricles. Furthermore, glasses wearers occasionally describe having difficulties wearing a BTE processor and glasses at the same time.

1.6.3 Current Sound Processors

Each CI manufacturer has its own sound processors and implants, which are not compatible with the systems of other manufacturers.

▶ An implant and a sound processor from two manufacturers cannot be combined. Likewise, patients cannot exchange sound processors among themselves. For bilaterally supplied patients who wear two sound processors from the same manufacturer, there is therefore no risk that accidentally swapping the sound processors will lead to discomfort.

Due to technical advancements, manufacturers introduce new sound processors at intervals of a few years. In the case of a surgical resupply, the latest sound processor model is always delivered. Repairs are made possible for older models for several years. If a model is so outdated that no spare parts are being produced anymore, an upgrade to the current sound processor is made at the latest at this point. In Germany, the cost coverage for the latest sound processor model is applied for at the health insurance company.

The CI manufacturers strive to maintain the compatibility of the implants with the latest generations of sound processors in the long term, so that patients with older implants can also benefit from the new technologies of the current sound processors. All available CI manufacturers currently offer a BTE processor, as well as the possibility of an EAS supply. Cochlear® and MED-EL each also have a model of a single-unit processor in their portfolio.

The constant development of new sound processor models and the regular technical adjustments in the clinic lead to a variety of individual supplies. For therapy, the specific supply parameters should therefore be asked for from the patient or the follow-up clinic. Further information can be found in Sect. 3.4 with hints and explanations on the use of the connectivity options of the individual manufacturers in therapy.

1.7 Opportunities in the Fitting of Sound Processors

Wiebke Rötz

The process of adjusting a CI is referred to as "fitting," and implementation requires special training from all manufacturers. In CI-supplying institutions, this task is primarily the responsibility of the audiological department staff. Initially, these are CI-specialized audiologists. Furthermore, hearing technicians and medical-technical assistants (of functional diagnostics) carry out adjustments after completing training. Always under the condition of specialization and participation in training, in other facilities (e.g., outpatient or inpatient rehab centers), also members of other professional groups (e.g., hearing aid acoustician or speech and language therapists) do fittings (DGHNO-KHC e.V. 2020, 52f.). In addition to the audiologists, regardless of the job title, we speak of CI technicians.

As part of the long-term follow-up care, after completing basic and follow-up therapy, appropriately trained and CI manufacturer-trained hearing aid acousticians can take over regular CI fittings. These are always done in consultation with the CI-supplying clinic (DGHNO-KHC e.V. 2020, 49 f.).

In the technical adjustment, the patient's sound processor is programmed. The stimulation by the implant is carried out according to the stored settings. The special possibilities and the handling in the fitting of a sound processor depend on the current software of the respective CI manufacturer (Target CI 1.0.20 from AB, Custom Sound 6.1 from Cochlear®, Maestro 9.0 from MED-EL, and Genie Medical CI from Oticon Medical).

Moreover, they are so variable that a comprehensive representation at this point is not possible. Therefore, we will focus on the parameters that are most significant for therapy. They can be roughly divided into sound-independent and sound-altering possibilities.

In order to reprogram the sound processor, the CI technician connects it to the software. As a rule, the transmission is done via a cable connection. Some manufacturers offer a wireless connection.

1.7.1 Sound-Independent Possibilities

After the sound processor has been connected, a brief check of the implant is carried out first. Within a few seconds, the electrodes are checked for their basic functionality. Afterwards, there is the possibility to gain insight into the wearing time and, with some manufacturers, to receive a situation analysis. This way, the CI technician learns whether the CI has been worn long enough attached to the head and, in some cases, can see how often a patient stayed in a quiet or noisy environment and for what period of time speech was heard. The less often a patient uses his sound processor, the slower the habituation to the CI system progresses.

In addition, the CI technician can determine within which framework the patient can change their own setting. This mainly concerns the change in volume across the entire frequency range, as well as the sensitivity with which the microphones should pick up the ambient noise.

In addition, further functions such as a slow automatic increase in volume after switching on the sound processor or the use for inductive hearing can be activated. These details are so individually different that there should always be an exchange between the CI technicians and therapists.

1.7.2 Sound-Altering Opportunities

In the initial fitting, a speech processing strategy is determined first, i.e., according to which rules the sound processor should process the recorded speech signal. Normally, the manufacturer sets a standard that is only changed if special conditions exist or arise in the fitting process. The reconfiguration of this strategy happens rather infrequently, but when it does, it is accompanied by a significant change in sound, which is why the CI technician should always inform the therapist. This may result in a change in the difficulty level of the exercises performed in therapy.

Both in the initial fitting and in the subsequent fittings, the main focus is on setting an optimal dynamic range. This describes the range in which the CI picks up and processes sounds. This range is limited by the hearing threshold (T-level) and the threshold of comfortable loudness, which is colloquially also referred to as volume (M- or C-level). The implants of each manufacturer have a set number of electrodes, which are accordingly attached to the electrode array of the implant. The T- and C-levels can be set for each of these electrode contacts.

Some manufacturers prescribe the setting of the T-levels, while others determine them individually. For this, the patient must indicate when they start to hear a tone or can no longer hear it. For the optimization of the C-levels, the intensity of the presented tone is increased until the patient perceives it as pleasantly and powerfully loud. For this part of the fitting, the feedback of the therapist is also relevant (Sect. 5.3). The C-levels are used to increase or decrease the intensity of individual frequency ranges.

Sometimes individual electrodes are switched off, which can have many different reasons. An increasing number of switched-off electrodes leads to stronger changes in sound. For example, there may be a short circuit or an implant defect, or the patient reports an unpleasant auditory impression. Furthermore, there is the possibility of a partial insertion of the electrode array, in which case the non-inserted electrodes are also switched off.

Also relevant for therapy are the various programs that can be stored on the sound processor. Each program can contain a completely individual setting of the aforementioned parameters or have various specifications of additional processing of the incoming signal based on the same setting. This means that filter functions such as wind noise suppression or the lowering of certain tones can be stored, or directional characteristics, which are supposed to ensure that sound is preferably picked up from certain directions in noisy environments (cf. Müller-Deile 2009, pp. 22–27; Adunka and Kiefer 2005).

1.7.3 Transmitted Frequency Ranges

A CI is primarily intended to make speech audible again. For this, the range in which speech occurs must be picked up by the sound processor and transmitted by the implant.

Fant (2004, p. 4) already attempted a schematic representation of Swedish consonants and vowels in the 1950s. The resulting shape of the speech field resembles a banana, which is why the representation of the speech sounds is often referred to as the "speech banana." Fant's original representation and derived speech fields for other languages are still valid and form the basis for the setting of various hearing systems. This can certainly be viewed critically. Steffens (2016) criticized, among other things, that only individual speech sounds, spoken by a few Swedish men, form the basis for the assignment. Because the speech sounds were not taken from a natural flow of speech, there is a deviating volume of the speech sounds, which does not correspond to the intensity of the speech sounds in spoken language.

▶ **Tip** In "Die 'Sprachbanane' repräsentiert nicht die normallaute Sprache" (English: "The 'Speech Banana' does not represent normal loud speech"), Steffens presents a corrected version of Fant's original proposal of the speech range.
    https://doi.org/10.1055/s-0042-105335

The main speech sound area, in which most of the relevant linguistic components are also located in German, ranges between 30 and 60 dB HL and between 300 and 4000 Hz (Kompis 2016, p. 101). This area is depicted in the pure tone audiogram. However, the entire speech sound range extends over a larger area, so that some linguistic information already occurs from 15 to 20 dB HL and between 125 and 8000 Hz (Steffens 2016). In this area, sound processors can pick up speech sounds, but how this is transmitted and perceived is a question of fitting and training.

In order to pass on insights from therapy to the CI technician, both sides must have an idea of which sound lies in which frequency range. This means for therapists that they should best refer to the naming of individual speech sounds or broader frequency ranges in their feedback for the CI fitting.

Basically, a distinction must be made between vowels and consonants. Vowels can be particularly well characterized by their formants (Sendlmeier and Seebode year unknown), which is more difficult with consonants.

Classification of frequency ranges using the example of the German language

- Low tone range with fundamentals: <250 Hz
- Middle tone ranges with overtones of vowels and other consonants: 250–4000 Hz
- High consonants: ≥4000 Hz (Lehnhardt 2009, p. 147)

Table 1.1 Classification of consonants into frequency ranges using the example of the German language

Frequency range	Voiced	Voiceless
Low frequency (125–500 Hz)	[b, v, m, n, l, z, ʒ, j, ŋ]	[ʁ, x]
Mid frequency (500–4000 Hz)	[g]	[ʃ, h, p, t, k, ç]
High frequency (4000–8000 Hz)		[s, f]

Generally speaking, the vowels extend over the low to mid-frequency range, while the consonants require a more individual assignment.

In order to divide the consonants into low-, mid-, and high-frequency speech sounds and thus be able to make more specific statements for the CI fitting, the division of the low tone range from <250 Hz made by Lehnhardt was changed to <500 Hz, and in Table 1.1 an approximate classification of the consonants into the individual frequency ranges was made using various speech bananas (Fant 2004; Klangpornkun et al. 2013; MED-EL 2022a).

Literature

Adunka, O.; Kiefer, J. (2005): Wie funktioniert der Sprachprozessor von Cochlea-Implantaten? In: Laryngo-Rhino-Otologie 84 (11), S. 841-50. DOI: https://doi.org/10.1055/s-2005-870454

Advanced Bionics (2021): Produktkatalog. Naída CI M & Sky CI M Soundprozessorn und Zubehör. Online verfügbar unter https://www.advancedbionics.com/content/dam/advanced-bionics/Documents/Regional/DE/Produkte-DE/Na%C3%ADda/NaidaCI-M/028-N091-01_Rev%20B_Marvel%20CI%20Product%20Catalogue_DE_A4_web.pdf, zuletzt geprüft am 17.02.2022

Advanced Bionics (2022): Advanced Bionics-Unternehmensgeschichte. Online verfügbar unter https://www.advancedbionics.com/de/de/home/about-us/history.html#, zuletzt geprüft am 17.02.2022

Arndt, S. et al. (2011): Unilateral deafness and cochlear implantation. Audiological diagnostic evaluation and outcomes. In: HNO 59(5): S. 437-46, Freiburg, Germany

Aschendorff, A.; Klenzner, T.; Laszig, R. (2005): Deafness after Bacterial Meningitis. An Emergency for Early Imaging and Cochlear Implant Surgery. In: Otolaryngology-Head and Neck Surgery 133 (6), S. 995–996. https://doi.org/10.1016/j.otohns.2005.03.036

Aschendorff, A.; Gollner, K.; Maier, W.; Beck, R.; Wesarg, T.; Kröger, S. et al. (2009): Technologisch-chirurgischer Fortschritt bei der Cochlear Implantation. In: Cochlear Implant heute, S. 39–46, Berlin, Heidelberg: Springer Berlin Heidelberg

Basta, D. (2009): Perioperatives Monitoring objektiv-audiologischer Daten im Rahmen der Cochlear-Implant-Versorgung. In: Ernst, Battmer, Todt (2009): Cochlear Implant heute, S. 31, Springer

Battmer, R.-D. (2009): 25 Jahre Cochlear-Implantat in Deutschland-eine Erfolgsgeschichte mit Perspektiven. Indikationserweiterung, Reliabilität der Systeme, In: Ernst, Battmer, Todt (2009): Cochlear Implant heute, S. 1-9, Springer

Bertram, B. (1991): Rehabilitation von Kindern mit einem Cochlear Implant. In: Lehnhardt E., Bertram, B. (Hrsg.) (1991): Rehabilitation von Cochlear Implant Kindern. S 63-103, Springer

Bertram, B. (1992): Cochlear Implant Versorgung ertaubter und taubgeborener Kinder an der HNO-Klinik der MHH und am Cochlear Implant Centrum Hannover (CIC). In: Plath P. (Hrsg.) (1992): Materialsammlung vom 6. Multidisziplinären Kolloquium der Geers-Stiftung, Schriftenreihe, Bd. 9. S. 109-116

Büchner, A.; Gärtner, L. (2017): Technische Entwicklungen bei Cochleaimplantaten. Stand der Technik. In: HNO 65 (4), S. 276–289. https://doi.org/10.1007/s00106-017-0339-7

Clark, G. M. et al. (1978). A multiple-electrode cochlear implant. In: Journal of the Otolaryngological Society of Australia, 4(3), S. 209

Cochlear (2021): Langjährig bewährt. Unsere Geschichte. Online verfügbar unter https://www.cochlear.com/de/de/about-us/proven-over-time, zuletzt geprüft am 23.02.2022

Demant (2022): Unsere Geschichte. Online verfügbar unter https://www.demant.com/ch-de/about/our-history, zuletzt geprüft am 25.02.2022

DGHNO-KHC e.V. (2020): S2K-Leitlinie. Cochlea-Implantat Versorgung: AWMF-Register (017/071)

Diller, G. (1997): Hören mit einem Cochlear-Implant. Eine Einführung. 2., veränd. Aufl. Heidelberg: Winter Programm Ed. Schindele

Ernst, A.; Todt, I. (2009): Die Entwicklung minimal-invasiver chirurgischer Verfahren zur Cochlear-Implant-Versorgung. In: Cochlear Implant heute. Berlin, Heidelberg: Springer Berlin Heidelberg, S. 47–52

Fant, G. (2004): Speech acoustics and phonetics. Selected writing. Kluwer Academic. Dordrecht: Kluwer Academic Publishers

Hamburger Morgenpost (1957): Titelseite, 17.08.1957

Klangpornkun, N.; Onsuwan, C.; Tantibundhit, C. (2013): Predictions from "speech banana" and audiograms. Assessment of hearing deficits in Thai hearing loss patients. In: The Journal of the Acoustical Society of America

Kompis, M. (2016): Audiologie. 4., vollständig überarbeitete Neuauflage. Bern: Hogrefe

Kramme, R. (2011): Medizintechnik. Berlin, Heidelberg: Springer Berlin Heidelberg

Laszig, R. (1993): First Brain Stem Implant in Europe (Auditory brain stem implant). Otolaryngol Head Neck Surg 111(1), S. 150-1

Laszig, R., Aschendorff, A., Stecker, M., Müller-Deile, J. et al. (2004): Benefits of bilateral electrical stimulation with the nucleus cochlear implant in adults. 6-month postoperative results. Otol Neurotol. 25(6): S. 958-68

Laubert, A. (1986): NUCLEUS – und alternative Systeme. In: Lehnhardt. E., Hirshorn, M. S. (Hrsg.) (1986): Cochlear Implant, Eine Hilfe für beidseitig Taube, S. 108-109, Springer Verlag

Lehnhardt, E. (1993): Intracochlear placement of cochlear implant electrodes in soft surgery technique. HNO 41 (7); S. 356-9, In: Ernst, Battmer, Todt (2009): Cochlear Implant heute, S. 1-3, Springer

Lehnhardt, E. (1998): Entwicklung des Cochlea Implantats und das Cochlea-Implantat Projekt Hannover, In: T. Lenarz (Hrsg.) (1998): Cochlea Implantat, S. 1, 2, 4-6, Springer

Lehnhardt, E. (2009) Sprachaudiometrie In: Lehnhardt E., Laszig, R. (Hrsg.) (2009): Praxis der Audiometrie, 9.vollständig überarbeitete Auflage, S. 147. Georg Thieme Verlag, Stuttgart. New York

Lenarz, T. (2017): Cochlear Implant – State of the Art. In: Laryngo-Rhino-Otologie 96 (S 01), S. 123-151. DOI: https://doi.org/10.1055/s-0043-101812

Leung, J.; Wang, N.-Y.; Yeagle, J. D.; Chinnici, J.; Bowditch, S.; Francis, H. W.; Niparko, J. K. (2005): Predictive models for cochlear implantation in elderly candidates. In: Archives of otolaryngology-head & neck surgery 131 (12), S. 1049–1054. DOI: https://doi.org/10.1001/archotol.131.12.1049

MED-EL (2021): Diese Elektrode gibt Arzneistoffe frei. In: Schnecke, Nr. 112/ 32. Jahrgang, S. 8

MED-EL (2022a): Das Audiogramm. Normales Hören. Online verfügbar unter https://www.medel.com/de/about-hearing/audiogram, zuletzt geprüft am 27.03.2022

MED-EL (2022b): Meilensteine. Online verfügbar unter https://www.medel.com/de/about-medel/our-history, zuletzt geprüft am 25.02.2022

MED-EL (2022c): RONDO 3 Audioprozessor. Produktkatalog. Online verfügbar unter https://www.medel.com/de/hearing-solutions/accessories/product-catalogue, zuletzt geprüft am 25.02.2022

MED-EL (2022d): SONNET 2 Audioprozessor. Produktkatalog. Online verfügbar unter https://www.medel.com/de/hearing-solutions/accessories/product-catalogue, zuletzt geprüft am 25.02.2022

MED-EL (2022e): Synchrony 2 Cochlear Implant. Made for Exceptional Performance. Online verfügbar unter https://sf.cdn.medel.com/docs/librariesprovider2/product/synchrony2/27304ce_r4_0-synchrony2implantfs-web.pdf?sfvrsn=3a799f42_2, zuletzt geprüft am 25.02.2022

Medical EXPO (2024): Nurotron®. Online verfügbar unter https://www.medicalexpo.de/prod/hangzhou-nurotron-biotechnology/product-74856-475234.html, zuletzt geprüft am 30.04.2024

Müller, J., Schoen, F., Helms, J. (2000): Bilateral Cochlear Implant – new aspects for the future? Adv Otorhinolaryngol. 57: 22-7, Würzburg

Müller-Deile, J. (2009): Verfahren zur Anpassung und Evaluation von Cochlear-Implant-Sprachprozessoren. Zugl.: Oldenburg, Univ., Dissertation 2008. 1. Aufl. Heidelberg: Median-Verlag von Killisch-Horn

Müller-Deile, J., Laszig, R. (2009) Audiometrie und Cochlear Implant In: Lehnhardt E., Laszig, R. (Hrsg.) (2009): Praxis der Audiometrie, 9.vollständig überarbeitete Auflage, S. 257. Georg Thieme Verlag, Stuttgart. New York

Müller, J. (2021): Bilateral: Mit dem Zweiten hört man besser, Schnecke, Nr.113/ 32. Jahrgang, S. 36-44

Oticon Medical (2015): Neuro Zti-Cochlea-Implantat. Bedienungsanleitung. Online verfügbar unter https://www.oticonmedical.com/-/media/medical/main/files/ci/products/neuro-zti/ifu/de/neuro-zti-instructions-for-use%2D%2D-german%2D%2D-m80402.pdf?la=en, zuletzt geprüft am 25.02.2022

Oticon Medical (2018): Neuro 2. Bedienungsanleitung. Online verfügbar unter https://www.manualslib.de/manual/403151/Oticon-Medical-Neuro-2.html, zuletzt geprüft am 25.02.2022

Rahne, T. (2021): Physikalisch-audiologische Grundlagen implantierbarer Hörsysteme. Über Energieübertragung, Ankopplung und Ausgangsleistung. In: HNO 69 (6), S. 475–482. DOI: https://doi.org/10.1007/s00106-019-00776-1

ReSound (2022): Bimodale ReSound-Hörlösung. Online verfügbar unter https://www.resound.com/de-de/hearing-aids/types/hearing-implant-hearing-aids, zuletzt geprüft am 23.02.2022

Robert, J., Briggs, S. et al. (2008): Initial clinical expierience with a totally implantable cochlear implant research device. Otol Neurotol 29 (2): S. 114-9

Schnecke (2018) „Ein gewisser Lautheitsunterschied", In: Schnecke, Nr. 99/ S.34 (versch. Quellen s. Artikel)

Sendlmeier, W. F. & Seebode, J. (Jahr unbekannt): Formantkarten des deutschen Vokalsystems. Online verfügbar unter https://www.static.tu.berlin/fileadmin/www/10002019/Forschung/Formantkarten_des_deutschen_Vokalsystems_01.pdf. Institut für Sprache und Kommunikation der TU Berlin.

Steffens, T. (2016): Die „Sprachbanane" repräsentiert nicht die normallaute Sprache. In: Sprache Stimme Gehör 40 (03), S. 105. DOI: https://doi.org/10.1055/s-0042-105335

Trieu, H. K.; Görtz, M.; Göttsche, T.; Osypka, P. (2009): Mikroimplantate in der Medizintechnik mit drahtloser Daten- und Energieübertragung. In: tm-Technisches Messen 76 (12), S. 578–582. DOI: https://doi.org/10.1524/teme.2009.0987

von Ilberg, C. et al. (1999): Electric-acoustic stimulation of the auditory system. New technology for severe hearing loss. ORL 61(6): S. 334-40, Frankfurt

Van de Heyning, P. et al. (2008): Incapacitating Unilateral Tinnitus. In: Single-sided Deafness Treated by Cochlear Implantation. Ann Oto Rhino Laryngol 117(9): S. 645-52, Antwerpen, Belgium

Wever, E. G., Bray, C. W. (1936): The Nature of bone conduction as shown in the electrical response of the cochlea. Ann Otol Rhinol Laryngol 45:822 In: Lehnhardt E (1998): Entwicklung des

Cochlea Implantats und das Cochlea-Implantat Projekt Hannover, In: T. Lenarz (1998): Cochlea Implantat, S. 1, Springer

Wick, C. C.; Butler, M. J.; Yeager, L. H.; Kallogjeri, D.; Durakovic, N.; McJunkin, J. L. et al. (2020): Cochlear Implant Outcomes Following Vestibular Schwannoma Resection: Systematic Review. In: Otology & neurotology: official publication of the American Otological Society, American Neurotology Society [and] European Academy of Otology and Neurotology 41 (9), S. 1190–1197. DOI: https://doi.org/10.1097/MAO.0000000000002784

Zeh, R. (2011): HNO-Krankheiten. In: Sozialmedizinische Begutachtung für die gesetzliche Rentenversicherung, S. 485-495. Berlin, Heidelberg: Springer Berlin Heidelberg

Needs of Patients in the Care Process   2

2.1 Importance of Hearing Ability and Hearing Loss

The sensory performance of hearing, as one of our five senses, is the acoustic bridge to the world around us. It allows humans to participate in the immeasurable variety of sounds, to absorb them, and to draw immediate conclusions for their actions.

But only the functionality and the interaction of all our senses allow us to recognize, experience, and interpret our world in all its diversity.

We can listen to the wind and the rain; the song of the birds delights us. Music can put us into rapture and trigger blissful feelings in us. However, it can also make us melancholic and sad. Emotional and prosodic components of the spoken language convey information about the emotional state of the conversation partner. If the sensory performance of hearing is severely impaired or even fails, the tragedy of such a dilemma becomes painfully apparent (see Bertram 2009).

2.1.1 Function of Hearing

The hearing organ is the ear (receptor), which makes changes in nerve potentials from the information contained in the sound (reception), which the brain can understand and process. But hearing also includes the unconscious processing of information in the various parts of the hearing pathway (perception) and finally the conscious evaluation of what is heard in connection with already existing experiences and the storage of new experiences (apperception) (Plath 1995).

▶ The ability to hear forms the basis of speech perception from an early age and allows us to conquer the inexhaustible richness of our mother tongue, which in turn is the basis of our interpersonal communication.

Acoustic signals warn of dangers and serve us for orientation in dangerous situations; music can enchant us. Even in the dark or over greater distances, we can receive acoustic information with the help of this sensory performance.

To the one who listens, it is also given to listen attentively and concentratedly to his interlocutor, but also to listen beyond what he says. The judge can listen to the defendant—whether he hears him is a completely different matter. Nevertheless, one can also mishear or even ignore what has been said.

The categories of listening say something about the relationships of the communicators to each other—be it participation, interest, ignorance, familiarity, social proximity, or rejection (cf. Richtberg 1990, 16).

Additional information is conveyed to the communication partners, among other things, by facial expressions, gestures, speech rhythm, and speech articulation as well as speech speed.

R. Jütte (2006) refers to the philosopher and music theorist Adorno, who distinguishes different types of listening: "Expert listening, good listening, educational listening, emotional listening, 'resentment listening' (as is supposed to be typical for lovers of Bach music), entertainment listening and simultaneous listening."

All of this seems to happen effortlessly as long as the sound recording is not disturbed. Hearing impairment in varying degrees is considered the most common congenital sensory deficit in humans. In Germany alone, about 15 million people of all age groups are affected.

"Hearing, of course, presupposes an intact sensory apparatus in the inner ear. But on the other hand, it also indispensably relies on the brain's ability to analyze and utilize the messages from the ear about sound stimuli or speech sounds immediately, in real time. This analytical performance of the brain is immense. Yes, since the inner ear recodes the sound or speech stimuli, recodes them into a sequence of signals that the brain can read, one could even say, 'We do not hear with our ears, we hear with our brain'" (Klinke 2006).

In this process, the CI takes over the function of the no longer functioning hearing sensory cells and transmits the speech sound converted into electrical signals via the auditory nerve to the brain. This alone is responsible for performing the sound analysis, deciphering and evaluating the semantic content of what is heard.

This fact proves the impressive brain plasticity to adapt to functional changes and, in the event of inner ear failure, to convert the electrical excitation patterns imposed on it by the CI into sufficient speech understanding. An impressive ability of higher neuronal structures.

The serious impact of hearing impairment can be very well demonstrated, among other things, by the failure of the "cocktail party effect." A hearing person is still quite capable in difficult listening situations of concentrating on their communication partner and following the conversation, as they can largely suppress noise. This is difficult for the hearing-impaired. Therefore, understandably, he avoids such stressful listening situations. This poses the risk of increasing social isolation (cf. Kollmeier 2006).

People in all industrialized countries are exposed to a constantly growing noise pollution. Aircraft noise, traffic noise, and loud music in all possible habitats contribute to this situation. The sometimes increasingly loud, aggressive acoustic stimuli imply that after decades of such noise exposure, hearing damage is threatened. The number of permanently hearing-impaired adolescents has been steadily increasing for several years. The reason for this is frequent and loud music listening via headphones, in discos, or at live concerts. In addition to these stressful noise exposures, there are also those caused by work, increasing the risks for future hearing impairment.

In addition, there are diseases such as meningitis, Meniere's disease, or sudden hearing loss in severe form, traumatic effects, or even ototoxic drugs, which in the worst case can lead to deafness of the affected individuals and have catastrophic effects on their social structure and self.

2.1.2 Impact of Lost Hearing Ability on Everyday Life and Social Network of Patients

The effects of increasing hearing loss should not be underestimated. It is not just about a reduction in volume, but rather encompasses further functions of hearing, such as spatial and temporal resolution, a decreasing clarity of acoustic signals, and the ability for frequency resolution. Likewise, the ability to discriminate speech from background noise is reduced. In the case of mild to moderate hearing loss, hearing aids can somewhat compensate for this deficiency, but this impaired hearing requires increased physical and psychological effort in interpersonal communication for those affected. People with unilateral deafness face similar difficulties, as two ears are necessary to follow a conversation in a noise-intensive situation, for example.

If a person becomes deaf, for whatever reason, this means a profound disruption in their life continuity, which an outsider can hardly empathize with. The inner ear of the affected person, the cochlea, can no longer fulfill its actual function as a microphone for recording sound events and their transmission via the auditory nerve to the corresponding brain areas. The sensory hair cells are irreversibly damaged. However, the functions of the retrocochlear information structures remain.

For those affected with severe hearing loss, deafness, whether unilateral or bilateral, the world has suddenly become different. They see the vehicles on the street, but can no longer hear them well, cannot locate them precisely, or do not hear them at all. Also, the conversation partner is increasingly difficult to understand because background noise significantly impairs speech comprehension. If hearing fails, only the moving lips testify that the other person is speaking. And the once beloved music from the radio, the CD, the smartphone, or during a concert—now nothing, only silence or simply unsatisfactory, increasingly strange.

> ▶ Considering the functions of human HEARING ability listed by Richtberg, one can imagine what it means to be deprived of all these functions, such as

- "the alarm function of hearing the orientation function of hearing
- the communication function of hearing
- the social and emotional perception function of hearing
- the psychodiagnostic function of hearing" (Richtberg 1990, 18-23)

Such a severe loss of senses inevitably leads to far-reaching disturbances not only in interpersonal communication, but also inevitably to previously unexperienced strains in the social structure. The previously unburdened family and professional life experience a massive collapse, and the fear of an uncertain future takes hold. Fears of failure, constant stress, oppress the affected individuals sustainably, as they unexpectedly face insurmountable difficulties. Until the onset of deafness, the problem of hearing impairment was not or hardly dealt with. The individual's quality of life suffers severe losses, and a carefree life seems hardly possible for the affected person anymore. They must embark on a search for a new identity, and they find themselves immediately in a life situation that is irreversible and in strong contrast to the one they have lived so far. A painful, bitter loss of quality of life and hoped-for life perspective.

At first, they feel overwhelmed to reconcile with this oppressive and exhausting, as well as frightening, life constellation. And every new day confronts them anew with this dilemma. Famous artists such as Beethoven or Smetana reflect their grief, their dismay at the loss of their hearing, in their musical oeuvre.

Those affected often feel left alone and misunderstood in this fatal situation of restricted or lost hearing, where they would have needed human closeness. The danger is that they withdraw socially, become depressed, and even risk slipping into isolation. Self-esteem is severely impaired, they feel inferior, and their previous independence is affected because they increasingly rely on help. The skin has become thin.

The family and the social network are called upon to cushion the sudden "crash" and to search together for ways to solve it. And without question, those affected also need immediate attention, help, and support. They also need the assistance of proven experts.

The resilience of a person, their attitude towards their hearing impairment, and their availability of successful or unsuccessful coping strategies (coping behavior) ultimately decide to what extent hearing impairments "[…] allow a relatively unburdened life, in which happiness or unhappiness, success or failure, regardless of the hearing disorder, take their normal fateful course" (Richtberg, ibid., p. 6).

Another issue is the increasing aging of our society and the associated increase in hearing disorders in this age group. However, those affected often deny this fact. Rather, they blame their immediate environment for it, because it allegedly speaks too quietly or too indistinctly.

They want to avoid hearing aids because they are perceived as a blemish. The high redundancy of spoken language allows those affected to compensate for a deteriorating hearing for a long time. The consequences of such an avoidance strategy are well known and make it more difficult at a later stage, with increasing hearing loss, to provide adequate hearing aid. This also increasingly impairs speech perception and its processing in the brain, due to a late-onset auditory deprivation. Adequate acoustic stimulation over a very long period was no longer possible due to the increasingly severe hearing impairment. In the case of presbycusis, morphological and pathophysiological changes affect almost all structures of the hearing organ (cf. Federal Health Reporting 2006, p. 22).

"Losses of nerve cells were also observed in the ascending auditory pathway. Accordingly, presbycusis can be characterized by both an inner ear hearing loss and an impairment of neural processing, i.e., the nerve connections between the inner ear and the brain. These peripheral and central hearing losses add up to an increasing loss of understanding of words, especially in ambient noise, impairment of directional hearing, frequency selection, and independent binaural (dichotic) understanding. Complicating matters for the elderly are often declining cognitive abilities, typical are e.g. problems with short-term memory, word-finding disorders, and concentration problems" (Federal Health Reporting 2006).

This constellation has led to an increase in CI patients in this age group and is expected to continue to do so.

2.2 CI Indication: Changes from 1984 to 2020

Since the beginning of CI care, the **indication** has significantly expanded.

In 1984, only bilaterally postlingually deaf patients were supplied with a CI. They only received an implant in one ear. Extensive preoperative medical and audiological clarification was indispensable. The "differential diagnosis of inner ear or auditory nerve disease" was a necessary prerequisite for CI care. For this, elaborate examination procedures were available. However, it was not possible "[...] to make a quantitative statement about the auditory nerve function [...]" and to draw conclusions about the number of remaining "functioning neural units." It was assumed that 5000–8000 nerve fibers were a prerequisite for understanding speech with the CI (Laszig and Luetgebrune 1986).

However, practice showed that even after decades of deafness, "[...] there is still a sufficient number of functioning ganglion cells left [...]" that is sufficient for electrostimulation with the help of the CI. The original number of about 20,000 ganglion cells is reduced to about 10%. The central auditory system retains its basic functionality (Lenarz 1998).

Both the installation and the functional proof of the auditory nerve (N. vestibulocochlearis), the presence of microphone potentials, and the exclusion of usable residual hearing were decisive prerequisites for the CI care at that time.

After years of successful operations and impressive postoperative successes in understanding speech with the CI, severely hard-of-hearing patients were also included in the selection from 1986 onwards. The basis for this was the extent of single-syllable understanding, which, however, no longer enabled verbal communication with conventional hearing aids.

Emergencies were and are particularly considered to be children and adults who have become deaf after bacterial meningitis, as obliteration with subsequent ossification of the cochlea is to be feared. In relation to CI care, intracochlear ossification can prove to be a considerable complication of the operation, "and requires special surgical techniques" (Aschendorf et al. 2009). A rapid CI supply is strongly recommended. Children with severe inner ear malformations also belonged to this group.

From 1987 on, bilaterally deaf children were operated on for the first time. Due to the good results, CI care was also extended to children born deaf, with a tendency towards younger and younger children. In 1996, multiple disabilities in children were no longer a contraindication (Lenarz et al. 1996; Bertram 1996). As early as 1995, deaf parents showed interest in the CI care of their deaf children, albeit hesitantly (Begall 1995).

Bilateral CI care has now established itself as standard care for children with a medical indication and for adults from 2000 onwards.

The advantage of early bilateral CI care in children is obvious, as it prevents auditory deprivation and promotes the development of binaural hearing.

The risk of possible postoperative complications increases for these patients, plus there is a significant additional financial burden for the cost units. There are also consequences for postoperative (re-)habilitation in terms of the technical adjustment of two sound processors and for the postoperative speech and hearing therapy of the CI cared patients. This circumstance particularly applies to those who have received their second implant many years later and, due to this large time gap, show a discrepancy between both sides. They will find it significantly more difficult to process the auditory impression conveyed by both implants centrally. And it requires a certain period of getting used to it, as both sides are still unbalanced at the beginning of postoperative therapy.

The development of directional hearing in bilateral CI care for postlingually deafened adults could be facilitated insofar as already existing central nervous connections of binaural processing, which have developed and manifested during the time of normal hearing, are available.

▶ Since 2000, bilateral care has become the standard for adult patients.

The electro-acoustic stimulation (EAS), possible since 1999, contributed to the expansion of indications. So-called hybrid implants are used. They enable "in addition to a safe surgical insertion of the electrode array with preservation of residual hearing a later simultaneous use of sound processor and hearing aid on one ear [...]" as well as "[...] synergies between electrical stimulation of the auditory nerve and the simultaneous acoustic stimulation of the still functioning inner ear" (Aschendorff et al. op. cit. 44 ff).

Advantages are also "seen in the fact that the CI is not capable of transmitting frequencies below 250-300 Hz. In the frequencies below this limit, however, there is certainly information that contributes to understanding speech and listening to music. In addition, the preservation of hair cells could have a positive overall effect on the peripheral auditory system, as neurotrophic factors are produced there, which support neuronal processes in the peripheral auditory system" (Battmer 2009).

However, at the same time, the question arises over what period the existing residual hearing remains functional. If it is lost, a reimplantation would be necessary.

In 2008/2009, initial studies on CI care for single-sided deafness (SSD) and asymmetric hearing loss (AHL) were conducted. This was associated with the hope of restoring binaural hearing, achieving tinnitus suppression, and improving speech understanding in noisy situations. There was also hope to largely reduce secondary symptoms such as stress or headaches, social isolation, and psychological stress disorders. However, the indication can only be made when a "radiological diagnosis of the auditory pathway and consultation in the case of proven significant restrictions in everyday communication" has preceded it (see DGHNO-KHC S2k guideline 2020, p. 31 ff.).

In the case of central hearing disorders, caused by bilaterally nonfunctioning auditory nerves, central-auditory implants or brainstem implants (ABI, Auditory Brainstem Implant) are available. The electrical stimulation is intended to enable auditory sensations (hearing sensations) and understanding of speech at the still-functioning auditory core. "The indication range extends to patients with neural deafness or cochlear deafness, in whom a CI electrode cannot be effectively placed due to morphological peculiarities" (Guideline DGHNO-KHC 2012).

The guideline of the DGHNO-KHC for CI care in Germany forms the basis for high-quality preoperative diagnostics and preparation for surgery. At the same time, it defines the high demand for postoperative therapy for adults and children. A CI care based on this guideline guarantees that patients to be treated according to the latest scientific and technical findings.

2.2.1 Indications and Contraindications Today

The decisive and guiding factor for the current CI care in Germany is the S2k guideline Cochlear Implant Care of the German Society for Otorhinolaryngology, Head and Neck Surgery e. V., which was revised under the leadership of the Working Group of German Audiologists, Neurootologists and Otologists (ADANO).

The research results and the decades of experience in CI provision are incorporated. The following medical societies, associations, and working groups, which were able to incorporate their own findings, were involved in the development:

1. Working Group for Cochlear Implant Rehabilitation (ACIR)
2. Professional Association of German Educators of the Hearing Impaired (BDH)
3. German Federal Association for Speech and Language Therapy (registered association) (dbl)
4. German Society for Audiology (DGA)
5. German Society for Phoniatrics and Pediatric Audiology (registered association) (DGPP)
6. German Cochlear Implant Society (registered association) (DCIG)
7. German Society for Neuroradiology (DGNR)
8. German Association for the Hearing Impaired (DSB)
9. The German Society for Neuropediatrics has been asked to participate.

"The guideline 'Cochlear Implant Care' is committed to the ideal of a respectful cooperation of doctors, technical experts, audiologists, therapeutic professionals and patients' 'at eye level.' The target groups are all professions involved in the diagnostic and care process, as well as those affected" (ENT Cochlear Implant Care, Guidelines 2020).

It serves to ensure the quality of cochlear implantation and the postoperative (re-) habilitation phase at a high level. This is of particular importance as more and more ENT clinics in Germany are getting involved in this provision.

"The goal in adults is the restoration of hearing with cochlear implants when sufficient hearing for verbal communication cannot be achieved with conventional hearing aids, bone conduction hearing aids or implantable hearing aids" (Guidelines, p. 7).

The guideline "Cochlear Implant Care" covers preoperative diagnostics, indication, contraindications, the operative phase, basic therapy (initial adjustment phase), follow-up therapy (CI rehabilitation), and long-term follow-up care in children, adolescents, and adults. At the same time, the prerequisites necessary for the quality of structure, process, and results are described.

The indication for CI provision takes into account audiological criteria that lead to a significant improvement in restricted communication ability. This is also associated with the goal of regaining a high degree of social participation. All findings obtained in the preoperative diagnostics are taken into account for the indication for surgery. The indication is determined separately for each affected ear. The auditory nerve and auditory pathway must be proven to be functional. Bilateral provision should be aimed for if the indication is given for both ears. There is an urgent indication in case of suspected obliterating labyrinthitis (see S2k guideline p. 26).

The S2k guideline fundamentally distinguishes between children and adults due to the diagnostic possibilities.

In the case of CI care for adults, the guideline refers to the distinction of the following:

- Postlingually deafened (after language acquisition) adults with residual hearing
- Prelingually (before language acquisition) deaf adults
- Single-sided deafness (SSD), asymmetric hearing loss (AHL)
- Auditory synaptopathy/neuropathy (see S2k guideline p.26–32)

The exact indication criteria for the individual patient groups can be found in the guidelines.

The S2k guideline distinguishes between absolute and relative contraindications for CI care:
Absolute contraindications for CI care

- "Evidence of a missing cochlea or a missing auditory nerve.
- The patient's inability to participate in the overall process of CI care (including basic therapy, rehabilitation, and follow-up care).
- No possibility or access to initial adjustment, rehabilitation, or follow-up care (patient- or facility-related, see structural process)."

Relative contraindications for CI care

- "Middle ear infections (implantation possible after sanitation).
- Limited rehabilitation ability in CI care.
- Negative subjective promontory test depending on the results of further audiological diagnostics.
- Severe comorbidities that significantly impair the care process.
- Lack of evidence of the auditory nerve in imaging" (guideline p. 33)

An age limit for adults is only given if the conditions for a promising supply are not guaranteed.

2.3 CI as a Chance for a New Beginning

Without a doubt, severely hearing-impaired individuals see CI care as a great opportunity for a new beginning in every respect, a help to overcome the massive communicative barrier caused by deafness. One is back and expects a fundamental improvement in individual quality of life, associated with a new sense of self-worth and a liberating independence. This affects both the immediate family environment and the possibility of emerging from previous social isolation, rebuilding and maintaining cherished contacts with friends.

With increasing hearing ability and hearing experience, characterized by constantly improving speech understanding, self-confidence, and the courage to participate in life in the usual way, grow. This circumstance is also associated with the hope of many patients to successfully reintegrate into their professional lives to be able to provide. The existing social law regulations are intended to give those affected legal certainty and support where bureaucratic obstacles make occupational reintegration difficult.

The effects of a successful CI supply are not only to be reduced to the functional rehearing and understanding of spoken language itself, but rather, it is equivalent to a liberating blow from years-long burden or even tormenting acoustic isolation. This is how many patients perceive and describe it in conversations. They have moved closer to the complexity of the many possible sensory impressions of their immediate world. Habituated mistrust is gradually reduced, as one is acoustically involved in conversation rounds again and can better follow the content of the conversation.

The new hearing builds up lost security, gives new self-confidence, especially with regard to verbal communication—those affected can control their voice, through the now again possible auditory feedback. In many cases, this control will also improve the voice quality and articulation.

But being back at the old workplace for those affected also means facing new challenges. This is understandably not easy, as for various reasons, not in every case of CI supply, there is a satisfactory improvement in speech understanding. Especially in noisy work situations, understanding speech, despite technical additional aids, causes many patients problems. This circumstance does not remain without impact on communication in the work environment, as the colleagues assume that the returned colleague hears again as before. And so, CI users always have to justify themselves and explain their new, still unfamiliar hearing situation and ask for understanding. Such situations are stressful for those affected. Here, consideration by the normal-hearing colleagues, intensive education, and the creation of adequate working conditions for those affected are needed.

2.3.1 Individual Possibilities and Limits of CI Supply

A number of factors influence the postoperative success of a CI supply. Only some of them are mentioned in this article.

An important aspect of individual CI supply is the motivation, the goal setting of the patients, their perseverance, as well as their willingness to face the expected, not insignificant demands over a longer period of time. A good family environment and a stable social network are undoubtedly very helpful and motivating. There, one usually feels caught and protected. The closest relatives, good friends, colleagues, who stand by one's side in difficult situations with advice and help, provide security.

For older CI-supplied patients, their life situation often presents itself as much more difficult, as many of them live alone in a household. They suffer from their reduced conversation possibilities with familiar people or family members, as these often no longer live nearby. Often, the long-time trusted life partner has passed away. A circumstance that carries additional psychological burdens.

The experienced deafness has left deep traces in the self-understanding of those affected. This requires special confrontation with the unfamiliar life situation, and so it will not always be easy to motivate oneself anew and face the challenges of postoperative therapy.

Nevertheless, especially older patients perceive their CI supply as a blessing and as a good chance to break out of private isolation, as hearing with the CI now opens up the possibility of communicating anew with others and participating in life in a new quality.

2.3 CI as a Chance for a New Beginning

Years-long near-deafness, coupled with an insufficient hearing aid supply, will due to the long auditory deprivation yield lesser hearing successes and comprehension performances, likely due to the negative effects on the neuronal substrate of the central auditory pathway. Therefore, from a therapeutic point of view, a longer period of time is needed, as well as patience and constant encouragement of the patients to minimize or overcome these initial difficulties.

Experience shows that those patients who only suffered for a short term or only a few years from a severe and progressively deteriorating hearing loss in one or both ears, quickly increase their hearing performance supported by the CI. An adequate hearing aid supply at the beginning of the occurrence of a hearing disorder and its consistent use enables a permanent, albeit very limited, auditory stimulation and contributes significantly to minimizing auditory deprivation. And under certain circumstances, patients who have learned to decipher some language information conveyed by the hearing aid despite their severe hearing loss, benefit particularly from the CI supply.

The higher age of many patients has a limiting influence on the postoperative hearing ability with the CI, as in individual cases, cognitive restrictions may impair this development process. Limited neurophysiological and auditory physiological potentials, duration of deafness, and possibly existing central perception or processing disorders can reduce or even severely hinder postoperative success. In relation to patients threatened by dementia, the question arises, to what extent the sensory reprovision of acoustic events contributes to mobilizing new forces and enables them and encourages them to participate more actively in life again.

The CI imposes electrical stimulus patterns on the brain, which it must recognize and identify as language. A short period of auditory deprivation, good verbal competence, and an unimpaired learning ability of the patient influence the success as positively as a quantitatively and qualitatively unimpaired auditory nerve. A realistic expectation of the patients also has a positive effect on the subsequent therapy.

▶ An essential prerequisite for hearing and understanding speech with the CI is the optimal adjustment of the sound processors. It must exactly consider the individual physiological situation of the patients during the adjustment of the sound processors, in order to enable a faster and better habituation to the new hearing impressions conveyed by the implant.

Poorly adjusted sound processors result in unbalanced hearing, produce noise, and deprive the patient of important information that is no longer presented to him (Basta 2009).

It is also necessary to make the patient understand that the Cochlear implant is a sensory prosthesis with only a few electrodes. In comparison, the normal inner ear has 30,000 sensory hair cells. This clearly shows the limited performance of the CI.

Very echoing and high rooms, as well as a high noise level, significantly make spoken language difficult or even impossible to understand. The limited directional hearing with monaural supply also causes problems.

The different supply options also influence the postoperative speech understanding:

- Bilateral supply: two implants,
- Bimodal supply: a CI on one side and the supply with a conventional hearing aid or hearing aids on the opposite side, which are compatible
- Unilateral CI supply
- Unilateral CI supply: opposite side normal hearing (SSD patients)
- Provision of a hybrid implant for residual hearing in the low-frequency range

From an ENT medical perspective, there are additional causes that are highly likely to significantly impair the success of a patient with a CI. Baumann (2018) lists the following causes, among others:

- "Lack of development or only weak development of the auditory nerve
- Deafness after neurosurgical intervention (e.g., removal of acoustic neuroma, surgery on the facial nerve or on the cerebellum).
- Meningitis with subsequent ossification or obstruction with connective tissue of the cochlea.
- Advanced otosclerosis with strong ossification of the cochlea
- Severe traumatic brain injury with temporal bone fracture involving the auditory nerve/ facial nerve.
- Deafness due to damage to the central auditory pathway (stroke, brain tumor, accident, etc.).
- Strong softening of the bony shell of the cochlea in severe otosclerosis
- Psychogenic hearing loss, phonophobia
- Severe malformation of the cochlea."

Further influencing factors that affect success can be found in the cited article.

2.4 Right to Comprehensive Preoperative Information

Preoperative patient education is of great importance. It should provide them with comprehensive information and answers to all questions related to the operation. These also include information about financing and postoperative therapeutic measures, as well as about medical and technical follow-up care.

Such an information package builds trust and contributes significantly to the patient's decision-making process. At the same time, the scope and quality of the consultation reflect the competence and experience of the consultants and the CI-supplying clinic.

To feel understood and supported is a comforting, valuable feeling for the patient seeking advice.

Hearing impairment or hearing loss has direct effects on the social fabric of those affected, both in terms of further life management within the family and in the professional environment. They increasingly encounter difficulties, if not even misunderstandings. Accepting hearing loss and successfully shouldering the associated burdens requires enormous strength and unshakeable trust in oneself.

2.4.1 Trusting Relationship as a Basis Between Consultant and Patient

Richtberg (1990) sees the most common sequelae and accompanying symptoms of hearing impairment as "psycho-vegetative instability, social withdrawal and loneliness, self-esteem crises, depression, etc.".

Opening up to these burdens of the patients represents a considerable challenge for the consultant. If he approaches it with empathy, he is most likely to gain the trust of the patients. The conversation will not always run smoothly, as there are certain challenges related to communication with the patients. Under certain circumstances, significant difficulties may arise because they do not understand everything acoustically or in terms of content. Misunderstandings on the part of the consultant are also not to be excluded. In light of the recent coronavirus crisis and the existing obligation to wear masks, this problem becomes even more apparent.

Patients should not be pressured into a CI supply. They would rather have the assurance that their decision on whether to opt for or against surgery is at their own discretion.

Thus, the offer to be available for a second conversation at any time for undecided patients is convincing proof of trust and reflects the respect of the consultants for the personality of the seekers of advice.

Another trust-building offer is the possibility to have a conversation with patients who have already been provided with a CI, so-called patient mentors. They can report from their immediate experience about their decision-making process, as well as about progress, but also about difficulties in the postoperative process of their hearing development and the associated therapeutic measures.

Comprehensive information material on the different CI systems and their technical aids contributes to the completion of the information needs of those affected. In clinics, CI therapy centers, or even in outpatient therapy facilities, where it is possible to observe during postoperative therapeutic measures, this should definitely be made possible for patients.

2.4.2 Tasks of the Consultant in the Enlightenment Process

The consultants are obliged to inform about both the possibilities and limitations of the CI supply. This also includes pointing out possible postoperative acute or later occurring complications caused by the surgical intervention.

With the decision for a CI, patients, per se, also take the risk of a possible reimplantation. This could be indicated if serious technical defects of the implant result in a total failure and thus simultaneously the loss of clinical benefit. But medical reasons can also necessitate a reimplantation.

The possible risks or complications that can occur during the surgical intervention must be explained to the patients in understandable language. It is essential to distinguish unambiguously between possible technical defects on the one hand and occurring medical complications on the other.

Thus, early acute complications such as wound infections, as well as transient facial weaknesses or disturbances of taste functions, can occur, among other things.

Late complications that occur after wound healing has been completed include problems in the area of the skin flap or occurring facial nerve irritations, as well as infections of the inner ear. Similarly, there can be electrode extrusions and the formation of cholesteatomas in the area of the ear canal and the middle ear. Unfavorable local nutritional situations of the covering skin flap, additional other diseases, or manipulations of the CI user on the skin flap itself could cause late infections (cf. Lenarz 1998).

The experiences gathered over many decades in CI provision, as well as the constant technological and surgical improvements, have contributed to largely reducing possible complications (Ernst, Todt 2009). Nevertheless, this information is essential for the patients and is proof of meeting them at eye level. Many patients inform themselves very intensively on the Internet, in forums, and at patient meetings.

For those affected who still have very little residual hearing, the decision for a CI is particularly difficult, as they must fear the loss of their residual hearing due to the placement of the electrode array in the inner ear. They therefore weigh up the pros and cons of their decision very carefully.

Patients must be aware of the significant time commitment in the postoperative phase. Having hardly or not heard anything over a longer period of time also means auditory deconditioning. Therefore, it takes an appropriate amount of time before they get used to the new electrically imposed auditory impressions, in order to integrate them into the overall sensory activity. Learning to hear anew with the cochlear implant is a dynamic process.

If the hoped-for success does not materialize, this can lead to great disappointments. This point also needs to be addressed, especially since the immediate social environment associates great hopes with the CI supply and may build up considerable expectation pressure on the CI-supplied. That means an additional psychological burden for the CI patients. Many relatives assume that normal hearing is immediately restored with the activation of the CI system. They are not always aware that a number of factors can significantly influence the postoperative success, both positively and negatively. Consideration, sensitivity, and patience on the part of relatives but also colleagues at the workplace are indispensable.

Therefore, it may also be advisable to offer psychological support for the discussion of all pending questions during the decision-making process for both the affected individuals and their immediate life companions.

Explanations about the development of postoperative hearing with the implant are indispensable for the patients and meet with great interest. The unfamiliar auditory impression caused by digitized speech processing and the speech processing in the brain requires an appropriate time to learn. In this context, the patients also need information about influencing factors that could potentially make learning to hear anew more difficult.

When counseling deaf patients, sign language interpreters are absolutely necessary to ensure error-free communication. This is also important because in the deaf community, there are sometimes crude and completely misleading information and ideas about the surgical intervention. These are based on negative experiences made over 40 years ago with an implant with a percutaneous connector. Discussions with deaf people also show that it is sometimes difficult to counteract this misinformation and existing resentments.

Preliminary discussions with patients with a migration background also require the use of native language interpreters in the counseling situation. This protects them from misunderstandings and inaccurate ideas about postoperative hearing and the necessary therapies due to a lack of German language skills (Sect. 3.3.4).

The experience background of a clinic in the CI supply of severely hearing-impaired people and a convincing response to their individual needs is a measure of its quality and a trust-building factor in the context of preliminary information.

In particular, therapists are called upon to perceive the patients not only as objects of postoperative speech and hearing therapy, but rather to be empathetic and understanding companions to them.

Literature

Aschendorff, A., Gollner, K., Maier, W., Beck, R., Wesarg, T., Kröger, S., Arndt, S., Laszig, R. (2009): Technologisch-chirurgischer Fortschritt bei der Cochlear Implantation, In: Ernst, Battmer, Todt (2009): Cochlear Implant heute, Springer, S. 43

Basta, D. (2009): Perioperatives Monitoring objektiv-audiologischer Daten im Rahmen der Cochlear-Implantat-Versorgung, In: Ernst, Battmer, Todt (2009): Cochlear Implant heute, Springer, S. 4

Battmer, R.-D. (2009): 25 Jahre Cochlear - Implantat in Deutschland-eine Erfolgsgeschichte mit Perspektiven: Indikationserweiterung, Reliabilität der Systeme, In: Ernst, Battmer, Todt (2009): Cochlear Implant heute, Springer, S. 6, 7

Baumann, U. (2018): Warum ich? Gründe für Gelingen oder Nicht-Gelingen der CI Versorgung In: Schnecke, Nr.99/ März 2018/ 29. Jahrgang, S. 17

Begall, K. (1995): Versorgung Gehörloser mit dem Cochlea Implantat, Stiftung zur Förderung körperbehinderter Hochbegabter, Vaduz, S. 59–90

Bertram, B. (2009): Hallo, ich kann hören. Ein Leitfaden für Eltern und Therapeuten, Gefördert durch die Cochlear Deutschland GmbH & Co. KG und die Professor Ernst -Stiftung, 2. Auflage, S. 10, 11

Bertram, B. (1996): Cochlear Implant für mehrfachbehinderte Kinder – pädagogische Erfordernisse und Erwartungen, In: Diller, G. et.al (Hrsg.): Neue Entwicklungen in der Diagnostik, Therapie und Technik. 2, Friedberger Cochlear-Implant-Symposium, Friedberg

Deutsche Gesellschaft für Hals-Nasen-Ohren Heilkunde, Kopf- und Hals-Chirurgie e.V. (2020): Cochlea-Implantat Versorgung, S. 7 ff, 31ff

Deutsche Gesellschaft für Hals-Nasen-Ohren Heilkunde, Kopf- und Hals-Chirurgie e.V. (2012): Cochlea-Implantat Versorgung und zentral-auditorische Implantate, S. 7, 12

Ernst, A., Todt, I. (2009): Die Entwicklung minimal-invasiver chirurgischer Verfahren zur Cochlear-Implant-Versorgung, In: Ernst, Battmer, Todt (2009): Cochlear Implant heute, S. 47–52, Springer

Gesundheitsberichterstattung des Bundes (2006): Hörstörungen und Tinnitus, Heft 29, S. 21, 22

Jütte, R. (2006): Hörfolgen – oder: Die Kunst und die Macht der Geräusche, In: Lend Me Your Ear, Ausstellungskatalog, Kunstverein Bad Salzdetfurth e.V. (2006), S. 40, 41

Laszig, R., Luetgebrune, TH. (1986): Klinische Topdiagnostik der Ertaubung, In: Lehnhardt, E. und Hirshorn, M. (Hrsg.) (1986): Cochlear Implant - Eine Hilfe für beidseitig Taube, Springer, S. 1

Lenarz, T. (Hrsg.) (1998): Cochlea-Implantate – Physiologische Grundlagen und klinische Anwendung, In: Lenarz, T. (Hrsg.): Cochlea-Implantat, Springer, S. 15, S. 42, 43

Lenarz, T., Bertram, B., Lesinski, A. (1996): Cochlea-Implantat bei mehrfachgeschädigten Kindern Konsensuspapier eines Expertenforums am 6.3.1994 an der Medizinischen Hochschule Hannover, Sprache-Stimme-Gehör, 20. Stuttgart, New York. S. 175–180

Plath, P. (1995): Lexikon der Hörschäden (Hrsg.), S. 97, Gustav Fischer Verlag

Richtberg, W. (1990): Was Schwerhörig sein bedeutet, Schriftenreihe für den HNO-ARZT, KIND Hörgeräte, S. 2, 6, 16–23

Kollmeier, B. (2006): Cocktail-Partys und Hörgeräte: Biophysik des Gehörs, In: Lend Me Your Ear, Ausstellungskatalog, Kunstverein Bad Salzdetfurth e.V. (2006), S. 56

Klinke, R. (2006) Das Ohr – Funktionen an der Grenze des physikalisch Möglichen, In: Lend Me Your Ear, Ausstellungskatalog, Kunstverein Bad Salzdetfurth e.V. (2006), S. 23

Variants of Therapy

3.1 Concept Clarification

Various terminologies are used and sometimes used synonymously to describe the therapy of patients with a CI.

In principle, a distinction can be made between the therapy in which practice is carried out and the therapy that serves for consultation. Different methods are applied and information is conveyed in both forms of therapy, yet there are inevitably overlaps when considering the patient with a hearing impairment holistically. This is by no means to be evaluated negatively and offers the patient a high added value through more individual care.

In Germany, the form of therapy in which practice is primarily carried out is listed in the therapeutic catalogue under speech and language therapy. Only appropriately trained speech and language therapists may carry out and bill for these. In addition to this designation, terms such as hearing therapy, speech and hearing therapy, or auditory training have been coined, which are not protected terms but describe the aspect of exercise treatment better. As the term auditory training is most commonly used in English-speaking countries, this term is used in the following chapters.

In addition to auditory training, "audio therapy" has emerged as another field of activity in Germany. During audio therapy, people with hearing impairment receive extensive advice on content related to the topic of hearing impairment. The designation audio therapist is not a protected term. An exception is the title audio therapist (DSB). Only people who have completed the 1-year further education at the German Association for the Hearing Impaired (registered association) and have a corresponding certificate can call themselves this.

Both therapy areas are always taken into account within the speech and language therapy training as well as in the further training to become an audio therapist, but are weighted very differently. It should be mentioned that the auditory training content within audio therapy is only touched upon, as audio therapists are not allowed

© The Author(s), under exclusive license to Springer-Verlag GmbH, DE, part of Springer Nature 2025
W. Rötz, B. Bertram, *Cochlear Implantation in Adults*,
https://doi.org/10.1007/978-3-662-72230-5_3

to take on speech and language therapy tasks in the traditional sense. Within the framework of audio therapy, only accompanying exercises to improve speech perception can take place; a full-fledged auditory training treatment after CI supply cannot be replaced by this.

3.2 Audio Therapy

Therapy with a CI patient can never be reduced to exercise treatment only, i.e., auditory training. A person with a CI is always simultaneously a person with a hearing impairment. Having a hearing impairment has a comprehensive influence on the entire life, affecting private and working life on various linguistic and nonlinguistic levels (Diller 2009).

When attempting to classify a hearing disorder according to the International Classification of Functioning, Disability and Health (ICF), it becomes clear that not only are the "functions of hearing (sense of hearing)" affected at the level of body functions, but also various other restrictions exist, especially in the areas of environmental factors and activities, and participation. The subchapters Learning and Application of Knowledge, Communication and Support, and Relationships are just a few examples of this (World Health Organization (WHO) 2005). The extent of the effects only becomes clear to most people when they are affected themselves, have exchanged information with those affected, or have informed themselves in detail about possible consequences and accompanying symptoms (Sect. 2.1). A lack of understanding of the consequences of hearing impairment and the possibilities and limits of care on the part of normal-hearing people harbors a high potential for conflict and thus promotes a reduction in social participation (Braun 2016, p. 50).

In everyday life, hearing impairment is almost invisible to people who are not aware of the consequences of hearing impairment. Initially, impaired hearing attracts much less attention than a broken leg or a hoarse voice.

Logical conclusions about reasons for certain behaviors of people with hearing loss can be difficult to understand if you are unfamiliar with the subject. For example, if someone talks incessantly and the conversation is very one-sided, you might wonder why the person has such a need to communicate, and you may even find it uncomfortable or exhausting. For most people, the fact that someone talks a lot without a break is not a sign of someone being hard of hearing and just enjoying a break from listening, which they may need after many hours of high concentration. As a result, a person with hearing loss can, in the worst case, even stand out negatively due to various behaviors.

But it's not just unconscious behavior, but also consciously experienced situations that may have been humiliating, discouraging, or depressing, that occupy people with hearing loss. Patients often report in therapy about exhausting family celebrations where they mainly nodded and smiled nicely to hide their hearing loss, about situations at work where they encounter a lack of understanding from their colleagues, or the fear of developing dementia because they suddenly become significantly more forgetful.

3.2 Audio Therapy

When hearing loss or deafness is detected, a whole new world of care options opens up. In addition to the actual hearing device, there is a large range of further accessories. The offer ranges from smoke detectors for the hearing impaired to transmission systems for conversations or audio sources. In addition, people with a hearing impairment are entitled to "compensation for disability" (Braun 2016), which those affected often are unaware of and therefore require counselling.

- A physician can diagnose a hearing impairment, prescribe hearing devices, or even perform hearing-improving operations.
- Hearing technicians can select and adjust suitable hearing aids.
- Speech and language therapists can bring about improvements in hearing and understanding with hearing aids and CI through targeted therapeutic measures.

3.2.1 Task and Availability of Audio Therapeutic Offers

The only remaining question is who will take care of all other issues and questions relating to improving the individual participation of people with hearing loss or deafness (Braun 2016). All mentioned professionals are capable of providing advice on a small scale, but for comprehensive support, a further offer is needed. Audio therapy is able to close a large gap in care and services and to connect and supplement the involved institutions, such as doctor's offices, clinics, and hearing or therapy centers. Unfortunately, this form of therapy is not widely available. While audio therapy is always offered in inpatient rehabilitation for the treatment of hearing loss and deafness, availability in an outpatient setting is very limited. In addition, audio therapy is not yet covered by health insurance in Germany.

There are now various further and continuing educational offerings in the field of audio therapy, which differ greatly in scope and content. Providers are, for example, the European Union of Hearing Aid Professionals (EUHA) (2022) and the German Association for the Hearing Impaired (DSB) (2022). The EUHA's offer is exclusively aimed at hearing aid acousticians, while the DSB's further education can be completed by anyone with completed training.

> **Contents of Audio Therapy in the German Language**
> Further topics of audio therapy are listed on the DSB's page.
> https://www.schwerhoerigen-netz.de/audiotherapie

3.2.2 Audio Therapeutic Support by Speech and Language Therapists

When conducting an auditory training with patients, one cannot avoid dealing with audio therapeutic topics or at least knowing about audio therapeutic offers that one can recommend to patients. For this, therapists must recognize an audio therapeutic need and address it. In the best case, patients can then be informed about consultation and care offers such as self-help groups, counseling centers, or possibilities of inpatient rehabilitation. Especially, self-help for people with hearing loss plays a significant role in dealing with hearing impairment. Here, patients have the opportunity to exchange with others affected, as the social network often shrinks with increasing hearing loss (Montano and Spitzer 2021, p. 183). Self-help groups can then provide a protected space and a way out of withdrawal and isolation.

If a therapist specializes in the field of therapy after CI, further training as an audio therapist is useful and supports the therapist in better understanding and relating the consequences of hearing loss for the individual.

▶ Tip Contact points for advice and exchange for people with hearing loss in Germany
1. Local self-help groups
2. Participation counseling centers (in Germany, for example, EUTB®)
3. Resident audio therapists or related therapy offers (in other countries, also depending on availability)

3.3 Auditory Training

The term auditory training describes the actual exercise treatment that is usually meant when talking about CI therapy. The basic structure is the same as that of other areas of therapeutic intervention in speech and language therapy: After anamnesis and diagnosis, therapy to improve hearing and understanding takes place. The framework can vary depending on the institution providing the therapy. The content implementation does not follow a standardized therapy concept, which would be difficult due to the individual prerequisites and needs.

It is sometimes mistakenly assumed that after the fitting of the sound processor, hearing and understanding would be normal again. However, the brain needs time and practice to assign previously stored auditory impressions to the differently sounding auditory impressions with the CI (Hermann-Röttgen 2010; Diller 1997) and sometimes never-before-perceived auditory impressions. This performance is possible due to the brain plasticity, i.e., the ability to adapt to new sensory impressions and to change structurally (Tremblay 2007; Schwemmle 2012). To support and promote this process, therapy makes use of the principle of coarticulation. It forms the basis for all subsequent goals of the auditory training.

Principle of Coarticulation
Verbal spoken language comprises different speech sounds that can be combined according to certain language-related rules. However, not only are the individual speech sounds strung together and realized in the same way each time. Depending on the sound combination in which a sound occurs in a word, it is articulatorily adapted to the sounds immediately surrounding it. This process is called coarticulation, which is a subfield of the linguistic area of phonetics (cf. Fellbaum 2012, p. 94; Daniloff and Hammarberg 1973).

This means that a CI patient, for comparison with previously stored speech sound patterns, needs to perceive not particularly frequent individual sounds, but as many different sound combinations as possible. This is the reason why, to achieve the goal of improved speech understanding, practice should primarily include verbal spoken language and predominantly sound combinations.

3.3.1 Framework Conditions

The prerequisites for conducting auditory training must be considered, depending on the service provider, as these vary depending on the institution.

The current German guideline for CI care provides for both basic and follow-up therapy in the first 24 months after implantation, as well as lifelong follow-up care. These services should only be performed in hospitals or specialized CI centers (DGHNO-KHC e.V. 2020). However, in reality, this is not possible everywhere, as, for example, long distances between the patient's place of residence and the hospital or the patient's working hours and the hospital's opening hours are not compatible. Therefore, therapy also takes place with speech and language therapists in independent practice.

While the frequency recommendation for individual treatment in independent practice in Germany is one to three times per week with a duration of 30–60 min, the approach in hospitals and rehabilitation centers depends on the respective concept. The guidelines recommend a total of 40 therapy days within the basic and follow-up therapy, and then only one day per year during long-term follow-up care. If outpatient or partial inpatient therapy is not sufficient, there is also the option to apply for inpatient rehabilitation measures (Sect. 3.3.5).

> **Therapy Prescription for Independent Practice According to the German Remedy Catalogue**
> 1. Indication: disorders of speech in severe hearing loss or deafness
> 2. Remedy: speech and language therapy 30 min/45 min/60 min
> 3. Prescription quantity: one to three times/week

▶ For patients, the formulation "speech and language therapy" can sometimes be somewhat misleading. The presence of a CI does not automatically mean disorders of the verbal spoken language of the CI user. The decisive factor is the presence of a disorder in hearing and understanding spoken verbal language.

Anyone who conducts auditory training with a patient supports the goals formulated in the guideline

- Optimization of the use of the implant through the sound processor fitting
- Improvement of participation in society and in the working environment through verbal communication
- Long-term securing of the achieved goals

These are overall goals and initially mean for the therapist to check the regular fittings of the sound processor for their effectiveness and benefit to the patient and to help the patient become accustomed to hearing and understanding with the current fitting. On this basis, the therapist accompanies and supports the long-term improvement of participation. The concrete implementation is described in Chap. 5.

Optimal patient care requires close interdisciplinary collaboration between CI-technicians and therapists (Sect. 5.3). In a CI-supplying clinic with attached follow-up care, or a CI center, this exchange is much easier to implement due to the spatial proximity of all involved professional groups than between the implanting clinic and independent practices. Since practices are not considered in the guideline, there are no recommendations for this. To ensure the necessary exchange, simple solutions are needed. (cf. DGHNO-KHC e.V. 2020).

The following possibilities for exchange are conceivable:

1. Request an auditory training report
   This option should only be used if the report is guaranteed to reach the CI technician. Even if the transmission of information is one-sided and does not offer the possibility for immediate exchange, it is still preferable to a completely missing agreement.
2. Use a form for written information exchange, which, to maintain confidentiality and data protection, is voluntarily brought by the patient. A sample form is shown in Fig. 3.1.

> **Tip** The form: "Auditory Training Feedback for the Fitting of the Sound Processor" is available for download at https://link.springer.com/chapter/10.1007/978-3-662-65201-5.

3. Direct exchange between professionals
   This approach requires a high level of patience, but is very effective when used regularly.

   Direct exchange requires prior release from confidentiality at both treatment sites.

3.3 Auditory Training

Auditory Training Feedback for the Fitting of the Sound Processor

_____   _____
Patient's Name   Practice

Masking of the opposite ear during auditory training (multiple answers possible)
☐ deafness on the opposite ear (no additional masking)
☐ switching off the hearing system on the opposite ear
☐ leaving the switched-off hearing system in the ear (with a closed earmold)
☐ earplug
☐ capsule hearing protection
☐ noise on the opposite ear
☐ direct streaming from an audio source to the CI
☐ other: _____

Required volume during auditory training
program: ____
sound level: ____ / increased steps from the program's baseline setting: ____

Tested programs
program ____ → use/ functionality: _____
program ____ → use/ functionality: _____
program ____ → use/ functionality: _____
program ____ → use/ functionality: _____

Unheard or faint speech sounds
_____

Frequently confused speech sounds
_____
_____

Abnormal frequency ranges
☐ lows → abnormality: _____
☐ mids → abnormality: _____
☐ highs → abnormality: _____

Needed programs for continuing the auditory training
☐ louder exercise program
☐ program for: _____

Other observations and notes
_____
_____
_____

© Rötz, W., Bertram, B.: Cochlea Implantat bei Erwachsenen, Springer Verlag GmbH, 2025

Fig. 3.1 Form: Auditory training feedback for the fitting of the sound processor, W. Rötz

3.3.2 Live Voice Versus Audio Playback

The most natural form of communication takes place face-to-face (live voice). Not only can you see the person you are talking to and therefore include nonverbal parts of the communication, but it also enables good sound transmission and recording of the spoken word. If speech is heard through a connection between an audio source and CI, the sound quality always depends on the audio source and the transmission medium. Therefore, training in live voice is preferable to regular practice via audio sources. Another great advantage is the variability of the speech material. Digital auditory training used in therapy sessions has exercises up to word, at most sentence level, which significantly complicates the increase in difficulty at a certain point in therapy. In addition, the therapist loses the ability to adapt the spoken words within an exercise to the individual needs of the patient through predetermined speech material.

Nevertheless, training via a direct connection of the CI to the audio source offers some advantages for special requirements in therapy. Firstly, exercises with SSD patients are made possible without the healthy opposite side hearing along due to incomplete numbing. The direct connection ensures that the audio signal is only transmitted to the CI. This allows the therapist to draw more reliable conclusions for the fitting of the sound processor. This approach is also suitable for patients who can only provide uncertain information about possible overhearing.

Patients who have been hearing poorly for a long time and have become unaccustomed to many noises and volumes are often unsure and react sensitively to the sudden increase in volume through the CI. Through a direct connection, these patients can often tolerate the volume better and learn that an appropriate volume is necessary at the beginning of the adaptation process in order not only to hear, but also to understand speech. As soon as the benefit of the volume becomes clear to the patients, they can also better accept an increased volume in everyday life, so that they can switch to live-voice after a few therapy sessions.

▶ If patients wear compatible hearing devices on the opposite side, the audio signal can be transmitted to both sides via the additional accessory. In this case, the patient must switch off the hearing device on the opposite side.

The use of audio sources is also helpful in the areas of tones, melody, and music. However, the sound quality of the recording should always be checked by the therapist beforehand.

If you want to use audio sources in therapy, some precautions must be taken. First and foremost, the patient must have additional accessories that can connect with the audio source in therapy. In addition, there should be the possibility to connect not only the additional accessory but also the therapist's headphones. Otherwise, it is difficult for the therapist to check the patient's responses in most exercises.

▶ If an audio signal is split between the additional accessory and the headphones via an audio splitter, the transmitted volume is usually reduced and may have to be increased again via the audio source or the CI.

Which additional accessories patients get with their CI and how they can use them sensibly in therapy is explained in detail in Sect. 3.4.

3.3.3 Therapy via Video Chat

The increasing digitization in the field of medical care also makes digital therapy offers within speech and language therapy possible; the pandemic events of recent years have even made it necessary. Specifically in auditory training, it comes in addition that not every patient has a CI-supplying clinic nearby and therefore has to travel long distances for fittings and therapy. Normally, the clinic aims to carry out the therapy as long as the clinic offers auditory training in addition to fittings. This is not always possible for patients with long travel distances, obligations in work and/or family life, and regular auditory training. To reduce the number of visits to the clinic, therapy via video chat, for example, is an option, but the actual offer depends on the clinic.

Online therapy requires additional preparations. The most important prerequisite is to ensure that there are suitable terminals with which the therapy is carried out. These must be equipped with a camera, microphone, speaker, and possibly connection options for additional accessories. The therapist should urgently consider the position of the microphone. Depending on where it is located and how the terminal is positioned or held, this can have a significant impact on sound quality. In addition, a stable internet connection is indispensable, as well as the corresponding competence on the part of the therapist and the patient in dealing with the technology. Choosing a provider for video treatments is difficult due to the number of providers. Ultimately, data security must be guaranteed first and foremost, which must be checked individually for each provider.

Above all, online therapy offers flexibility in terms of time and location and may even be a more effective form of therapy for the group of SSD patients. SSD patients often cannot be adequately temporarily masking the ear on their normal-hearing side, which is one of the most important basic rules in auditory training (Sect. 5.1.2). Due to the direct connection of the CI and the terminal and the resulting inactivity of the speakers, exclusive transmission of the signal to the CI is ensured and listening on the normal-hearing side is excluded. Another basic rule is understanding without seeing the mouth shape. Whether the patient looks away cannot always be reliably assessed via the camera, but could be ensured by deactivating the video by the therapist.

▶ In therapy via video chat, the insufficient masking of the opposite ear can be circumvented in SSD patients.

There are no deviations in the structure of the therapy, but some special features must be considered when using materials and techniques to support the understanding (Sect. 5.2.1). Basically, any image or written material is rather difficult to use. This must be sent to the patient in advance. Although the therapist can share their own screen with most providers and make digital materials visible to the patient, this could be difficult as patients often use their smartphones for therapy, which has a screen size that is too small for many materials. If an initial letter or a selection of words is given as a visual supporting technique, this could be implemented via the chat function spontaneously due to the small amount of text.

▶ **Tip** In order not to lose valuable therapy time during online sessions, the use of technology should be tested in a face-to-face appointment with the patient in advance, and a telephone number should be obtained through which the patient can be reached in case of technical difficulties. For uncertain patients, the presence of a supportive person to set up the therapy session during the first appointments is recommended. This prevents overloading under unexpected circumstances.

3.3.4 Therapy in a Foreign Language

Due to various migration movements of the last decades, according to the "Statistische Bundesamt" (engl.: Federal Statistical Office) (2021), currently 11.4 million people without German citizenship live in Germany. Although the number of those who have little or no knowledge of German is not the same as the number of foreign nationals, it does at least provide an orientation for classifying the resulting difficulties in therapy. In addition to a few nonlinguistic exercise areas (Sect. 5.1), the language itself is mainly the therapeutic agent in auditory training. Therefore, the barrier should be as low as possible at the level of language competence. To date, there is no comprehensive solution for such patients in Germany, which means that, in most cases, the treatment goal must be minimized. This means that the primary aim is to achieve a satisfactory sound processor fitting. Support in the process of disability acceptance, towards the best possible communication in everyday life, remains difficult for the time being.

The therapist must first evaluate the extent to which patients have knowledge of German in order to assess whether therapy in German is at least fundamentally possible. Furthermore, the therapist must be able to distinguish when a patient cannot understand the language material due to a language barrier or acoustically. This can only be achieved through dialogue with patients and relatives and must be considered extremely individually. If a few words and simple sentences can be understood, this may be sufficient for the first therapy sessions. If this is not the case, there is the option to resort to bilingual therapists, interpreters, and translation apps.

The best options arise for patients in the care of a therapist who speaks the patient's language at a native level. However, bilingual therapists are an exception and are not available to everyone in their local area.

▶ **Tip** Every CI-supplying clinic should be aware of multilingual therapy offers in their area in order to be able to refer to them if necessary.

The involvement of interpreters can also be helpful. Regardless of whether they are professional interpreters or lay interpreters, their use must be critically viewed due to the lack of quality standards for the complex field of speech and language therapy (Scharff Rethfeldt 2017). In addition, the involvement of an interpreter always means a significantly higher concentration effort for the therapist, as interpreters usually do not have the linguistic knowledge necessary for the evaluation of sound processor fittings. With lay interpreters, such as relatives or friends, the involvement is additionally complicated by the fact that the relationship to the patient influences the type of translation (Merse 2020, p. 68).

The use of translation apps is similarly difficult, as these apps cannot yet replicate the performance of a native speaker. Nevertheless, the use of apps can support therapy to obtain rough information about the current sound processor fitting. From a study in which various apps were compared for their suitability for speech and hearing therapy, "Google Translate" emerged as the currently best option (Rötz et al. 2022).

3.3.5 Outpatient Versus Inpatient Rehabilitation

As already described in the framework conditions, the design of outpatient rehab depends on the follow-up clinic. As a rule, it normally starts immediately after the first fittings and takes place once or twice a week. Some clinics also implement follow-up care in the form of semi-inpatient rehab, for which the patients are on site for several days at a time at larger intervals. In the first weeks to months after the initial fitting, patients usually make the greatest progress, so that a good basis of understanding with the CI can be achieved on an outpatient or semi-inpatient basis. In terms of content, this usually involves a combination of regular fittings and auditory training, as also provided for in the guideline (DGHNO-KHC e.V. 2020).

In Germany, there is also the possibility of undergoing inpatient rehab in designated facilities. Authorization is usually granted for a period of 3 weeks. If a patient requires more time, the rehabilitation facility applies for an extension of the measure. In the analysis by Zeh and Baumann (2015), the average length of stay was between 4 and 5 weeks.

Such inpatient rehab is possible at any time, but it must be individually weighed for each patient when an inpatient measure appears most suitable. The decision about the timing depends on the general condition, the handling of one's own hearing loss, and the hearing test results with the CI. The more severely a patient is affected by the hearing situation and the less well they understand speech in the first few weeks, the sooner an inpatient rehabilitation program should be considered. Due to the implantation, inpatient rehab with CI is not automatically approved. Although in Germany there is an extensive legal basis for argumentation anchored in the SGB IX (Zeh and Baumann 2015), rehab must always be applied for from the relevant cost unit.

The most significant advantage of inpatient rehab lies in the therapy frequency and therapy variability. In addition to daily individual and group auditory training, there is an offer of regular fittings of the sound processor, audio therapeutic advice, possibly psychological accompaniment, movement therapies, instructions for relaxation exercises, and various information events such as lectures and communication groups. Thus, inpatient rehab offers a large number of ICF-oriented interventions, in which not only the improvement of language comprehension is pursued as an isolated goal, but also the confrontation with one's own disability and the individual support of this process.

3.4 Connectivity and Accessories

For people with a hearing impairment, there are various options for fitting additional accessories besides the respective hearing system. The function of such aids is to make acoustic signals more audible or perceptible to other senses (light or vibration) or to facilitate speech comprehension. During auditory training, patients can be advised or instructed to use these in their everyday lives. In some therapy situations with patients, it may be useful to use those accessories during the exercises.

If there is a particularly urgent and large need for advice, the CI-supplying clinic or the hearing aid acoustician can be consulted to find solutions quickly. Alternatively, it should be considered to discuss this topic as part of inpatient rehab. Here, audio therapists respond to every individual's needs and allow various accessories to be tested without obligation.

▶ **Tip** Information on additional technical accessories can be obtained, for example, from
- Hearing aid acousticians
- CI manufacturers for manufacturer-specific accessories (customer service or via the CI-supplying clinic)
- Online shops, which sell additional technical accessories
- Homepages and customer service of manufacturers of additional accessories

3.4.1 Categories of Technical Accessories for People with Hearing Impairment

3.4.1.1 Alarm Devices
In everyday life, we encounter many acoustic signals, which can limit accessibility for those with hearing impairments. Only when we deal with this topic in concrete

3.4 Connectivity and Accessories

terms do we realize how acoustically oriented people have designed their environment. For some signals, there is the possibility to amplify them or make them perceptible in other ways, e.g., vibration. Such alarm devices are offered by hearing aid and accessory manufacturers.

> **Examples of Components of Signaling Systems or Individual Devices with Light or Vibration**
> 1. Smoke detectors
> 2. CO-smoke detectors
> 3. Baby monitors
> 4. Alarm systems
> 5. Water level detectors
> 6. Doorbells
> 7. Telephone bells

▶ **Legal Entitlement to Smoke Detectors** In Germany, for a certain degree of hearing impairment, there is a legal entitlement to cost coverage for the provision of smoke detectors that can also be perceived by people with any kind of hearing impairment. Detailed information can be obtained from the respective health insurance company.

3.4.1.2 Telephones

Telephones for the hearing impaired represent a special group, as the alarm function and audio transmission overlap, as well as the offerings of cochlear implant, hearing aid, and other accessory manufacturers. Due to its additional high relevance in everyday life, a very large market has developed that should be considered separately.

During telephone training in therapy (Sect. 5.1.7), it becomes clear what needs the patient has when talking on the phone with the cochlear implant. Accordingly, it should be weighed whether the purchase of a new telephone or an additional accessory that is connected to one's own telephone is necessary.

> **Possible Features of Telephones for the Hard of Hearing**
> - Variation of the basic volume
> - Frequency-dependent volume setting (e.g., vary only bass or high frequencies)
> - Bluetooth capable
> - Induction capable
> - Audio jack for connecting to other transmission technologies
> - Loud signal tones

▶ Consultation about a suitable telephone or technology that can be connected to an existing telephone should always take place before patients turn to any electronics store. There, the offer is very limited, and often "hard-of-hearing telephones" are offered, which mainly have a higher output volume. This alone usually only slightly facilitates understanding on the telephone or not at all.

3.4.1.3 Audio Transmission

To support the transmission of speech and music, either from an audio source or via live voice, accessories are available from every CI manufacturer and many hearing aid manufacturers that are compatible with their own devices. Similarly, manufacturer-independent technology can be used via appropriate interfaces.

3.4.2 Transmission Paths

As in communication, the transmission of information via technical devices is also based on the sender-receiver model. The sender can either be a signal source (e.g., doorbell), a speaker, or an audio source (e.g., television). Corresponding receivers can be signal transmitters (e.g., flash modules) or the hearing systems (e.g., CI or hearing aid) themselves. Additional accessories for people with hearing loss can record the information from the sender and act as a new sender or transmitter/interface between the original sender and the receiver. Technological progress in this area now also makes direct connections possible, without such a transmitter.

3.4.2.1 Cable Transmission

A direct transmission from sender to receiver via a cable connection was standard for various additional accessories for a long time, before radio transmitters and wireless direct connections increasingly became more common. This type of transmission is almost only used for shorter transmission routes from the sender to the transmitter, although even here, in most cases, wireless transmission paths are possible.

Use of a Cable for Information Transmission

Television → cable → transmitter → wireless transmission → hearing system
Doorbell → cable → transmitter → wireless transmission → flashlight lamp
Mobile phone → cable → (older) → hearing system ◄

3.4.2.2 Wireless Transmission

Wireless connections between senders, transmitters, and receivers can be based on the various transmission possibilities of radio, infrared, and induction.

Infrared

When infrared is used, information is transmitted via infrared light, which can't be seen by the human eye. In everyday life, this is encountered in remote controls, for example. In the field of hearing support technology, infrared transmission is very rarely used. Since a line of sight from the transmitter to the sending device is necessary, this transmission route is rather impractical and therefore only suitable for activities where you move little, such as watching television.

> **Use of Infrared for Information Transmission**
>
> Television → cable → infrared transmitter → infrared transmission → infrared receiver (e.g., to hang around the neck) → wireless transmission → hearing system ◄

Induction

An inductive transmission is, simply put, the transfer of information via an electromagnetic field. Within a transmission system, an electromagnetic field must be generated by an induction loop and received by an induction coil. An induction loop can be laid in the room or worn around the neck in a smaller version. The induction coil is ideally located in the hearing system, but can also be installed in a device that ultimately transmits the information to the hearing system via radio. Synonyms for the induction coil are also the terms T-coil or telecoil. The induction coil must be actively switched on and off by the wearer of the hearing system. Opportunities for inductive hearing are provided worldwide, and inductive hearing with hearing systems is theoretically always possible regardless of the manufacturer. It then depends on the specific hearing system and if it's able to receive information via induction. Therefore, this technology is often used in public spaces, such as in cinemas, theaters, at reception desks, or in lecture rooms. An existing system is characterized by the pictogram of the crossed-out ear with a "T" next to it.

> **Use of Induction for Information Transmission**
>
> Microphone or speaker signal → cable or wireless transmission → induction loop in the floor → inductive transmission → hearing system with induction coil
>
> Microphone → wireless transmission → induction loop to wear around the neck with receiver for the microphone signal → inductive transmission → hearing system with induction coil
>
> Telephone with induction loop in the receiver → inductive transmission → hearing system with induction coil ◄

Since other devices or objects, e.g., fire-rated doors and generate electromagnetic fields, there can be disturbances in hearing if the induction coil is forgotten to be switched off or such objects and devices are in direct proximity. Patients often describe the interference noises as humming or buzzing.

Radio

Transmission of information via radio allows the patient the greatest freedom of movement and usually interference-free hearing. It is also almost always used in signaling systems. Since Bluetooth® transmission is usually used, there can occasionally be disturbances with, for example, devices in a neighboring apartment, but this is rather the exception.

This technology can be used particularly comfortably for audio transmission when the hearing system is directly compatible with the audio source.

Use of Radio for Information Transmission

Radio smoke detector → radio transmission → alarm clock with flashing light

Television → microphone compatible with the hearing system, which records the TV sound → radio transmission → hearing system

Mobile phone → radio transmission → hearing system ◀

3.4.3 Use of Additional Technical Accessories in Therapy

In everyday communication, patients are dependent on supplementing their acoustic understanding with additional information, despite being supplied with a CI. This can be obtained through "lip-seeing" (Sect. 5.1.2), observing facial expressions and gestures, and additional technical accessories. For optimal support, as much additional technology as necessary, but as little as possible, should be used.

The initial equipment that comes with a CI, which is paid for by the health insurance, always includes at least one additional technical accessory, which was selected in advance or a corresponding voucher. Each manufacturer has at least one device, or a selection, from which the patient can choose one. Not all options always serve to support communication. This makes it all the more important to discuss with the patient which technology would be of particular benefit to them (Braun 2016). This is usually taken over by the CI-supplying clinic during the first fittings. If an order has not yet been placed before the implantation because the patient was still unsure, the accessories can also be reordered from the CI manufacturer several weeks later.

In addition, patients have the opportunity to buy additional aids privately or to receive them after application via a cost unit such as the health insurance. Since the available product range of the individual manufacturers is very large and subject to constant development, the following will only go into more detail on how the devices of the initial equipment can be used in therapy.

3.4 Connectivity and Accessories

Advanced Bionics (AB)

> **Selection of the initial equipment**
> - Phonak TV Connector (audio streamer for the TV)
> - Phonak RemoteControl (remote control)
> - Phonak PartnerMic™ (remote microphone for distance communication)
> - Roger X with 02 license (Roger radio receiver)
>
> **Additional transmission options**
> - Induction coil in all sound processors
> - Direct transmission from selected mobile phones
>
> (Advanced Bionics 2021)

The PartnerMic™ can be used in therapy if it is necessary to maintain a certain distance between the patient and the therapist to avoid overhearing on the opposite ear. The PartnerMic™ can also be tested for everyday use.

In telephone training, the direct transmission from the mobile phone to the sound processor can be used, if this is possible with the patient's phone.

Cochlear®

> **Selection of the initial equipment**
> - True Wireless™ devices (Fig. 3.2)
> - Phone clip (connection to phones via Bluetooth®)
> - Mini microphone 2+ (clip-on microphone with audio jack, FM jack, and induction coil)
> - Audio Transmitter (TV streamer for transmitting the TV signal)
>
> **Additional transmission options**
> - Induction coil in the Nucleus®8
> - Induction coil in the Mini Microphone 2+
> - Direct transmission from selected mobile phones
> - Radio transmission via Roger20 radio receiver for the Nucleus®8 or RogerX receiver for the Mini Microphone 2+
> - Bluetooth® LE Audio for transmitting Auracast® Broadcast Audio
>
> (Cochlear 2024)

Fig. 3.2 True Wireless™ devices (from left to right): Audio Transmitter, Mini Microphone 2+, Phone Clip (images courtesy of Cochlear. © Cochlear Limited 2022. All rights reserved)

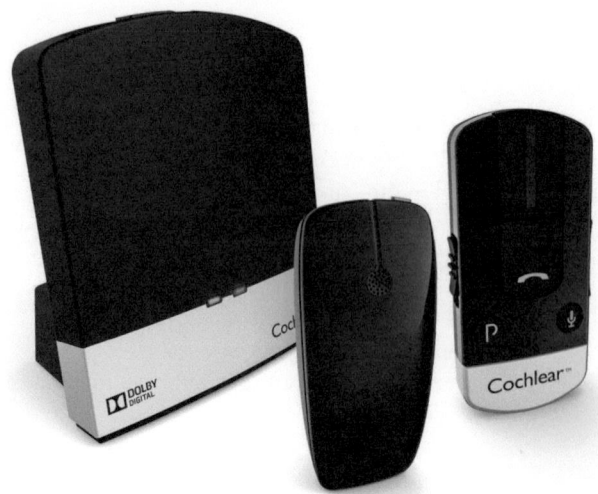

The Mini Microphone 2+ can connect the patient's CI to an audio source such as a PC or speaker, and auditory training can be carried out using it. A cable connection is made between the microphone and the audio source. This can also be practiced in the area of music listening via a direct connection. In addition, the therapist can use the Mini Microphone 2+ to maintain a distance between the patient and the therapist or to test communication situations in everyday life.

Furthermore, the phone clip and a possible direct transmission from the mobile phone to the CI can be integrated into telephone training.

MED-EL

Included in the initial equipment
- AudioLink with docking station (Bluetooth®-enabled device with audio jack and microphone for attachment Fig. 3.3)
- AudioStream battery sleeve for the SONNET 2 (Bluetooth®-enabled)

Additional transmission options
- Induction coil in the SONNET 2
- Induction coil module for attaching to the RONDO 3
- Roger21 receiver for the SONNET 2
  (MED-EL 2022a, b, c)

3.4 Connectivity and Accessories

Fig. 3.3 AudioLink with docking station. (Courtesy of MED-EL. All rights reserved)

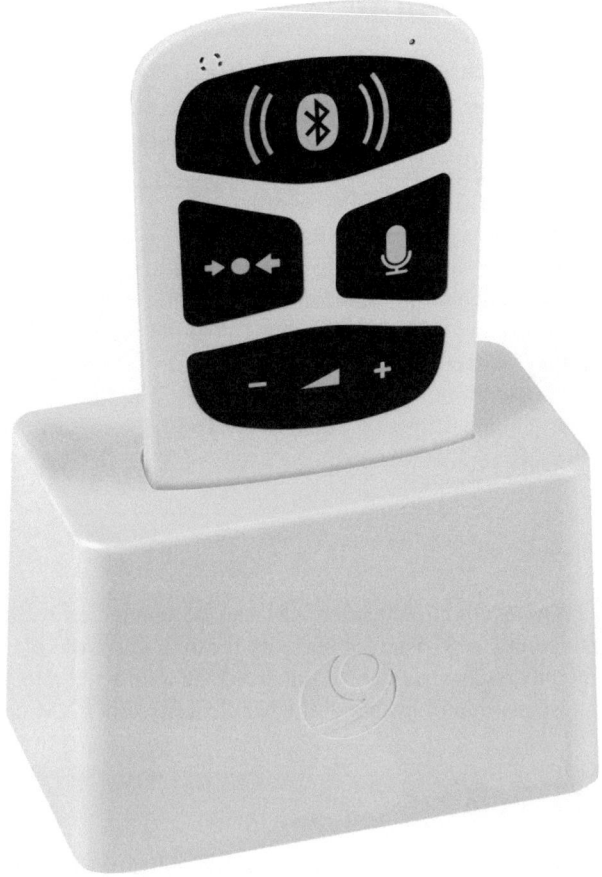

The AudioLink can be connected to other audio sources via a cable connection or Bluetooth® to use the audio transmission for auditory training. Furthermore, this can be practiced when training with music via a direct connection. In addition, the therapist can use the AudioLink as a microphone to practice even at a greater distance from each other or for everyday use.

For telephone training, both the AudioLink and the AudioStream sleeve (when supplied with a SONNET 2) can be integrated.

Oticon Medical (OM)

> **Included in the initial equipment**
> Medical Streamer XM (Bluetooth®-enabled device with microphone for phoning, audio jack, and FM jack)
>
> **Additional transmission options**
> - Induction coil in the sound processor
> - Devices from the ConnectLine series (must be purchased privately):
> - ConnectLine Microphone (lapel microphone)
> - ConnectLine Telephone Adapter 2.0 (transmission from the landline telephone)
> - ConnectLine TV Adapter 2.0 (transmission of the TV signal)
> - RogerX receiver for the Medical Streamer XM
> (Oticon Medical 2018, 2022)

The Medical Streamer XM can be connected to an audio source via cable or Bluetooth® and used for auditory training via audio playback. Furthermore, hearing melody and music can be practiced via a direct connection.

In the area of phoning, the Medical Streamer XM can be tested together.

Literature

Advanced Bionics (2021): Produktkatalog. Naída CI M & Sky CI M Soundprozessorn und Zubehör. Online verfügbar unter https://www.advancedbionics.com/content/dam/advancedbionics/Documents/Regional/DE/Produkte-DE/Na%C3%ADda/NaidaCI-M/028-N091-01_Rev%20B_Marvel%20CI%20Product%20Catalogue_DE_A4_web.pdf, zuletztgeprüftam17.02.2022

Braun, A. (2016): Cochlea-Implantat (CI)-Rehabilitation bei postlingual ertaubten CI-Trägern. In: Hörakustik (9), S. 50–52

Cochlear (2024): https://www.cochlear.com/de/de/home/products-and-accessories/cochlear-nucleus-system/nucleus-sound-processors. Zugegriffen: 03.05.2024

Daniloff, R. G.; Hammarberg, R. E. (1973): On defining coarticulation. In: Journal of Phonetics 1 (3), S. 239–248. https://doi.org/10.1016/S0095-4470(19)31388-9

Deutscher Schwerhörigenbund e.V. (DSB) (2022): Online verfügbar unter www.schwerhoerigen-netz.de, zuletzt geprüft am 12.01.2022

DGHNO-KHC e.V. (2020): S2K-Leitlinie. Cochlea-Implantat Versorgung: AWMF-Register (017/071)

Diller, G. (1997): Hören mit einem Cochlear-Implant. Eine Einführung. 2., veränd. Aufl. Heidelberg: Winter Programm Ed. Schindele.

Diller, G. (2009): (Re)habilitation nach Versorgung mit einem Kochleaimplantat. In: HNO 57 (7), S. 649–656. https://doi.org/10.1007/s00106-009-1922-3

Europäische Union der Hörakustiker e.V. (2022): Online verfügbar unter www.euha.org, zuletzt geprüft am 12.01.202

Literature

Fellbaum, K. (2012): Sprachverarbeitung und Sprachübertragung. 2. Aufl. Berlin, Heidelberg: Springer

Hermann-Röttgen, M. (Hrsg.) (2010): Cochlea-Implantat. Ein Ratgeber für Betroffene und Therapeuten. 1. Aufl., Stuttgart, TRIAS

MED-EL (2022a): Audio Link. User manual. Online verfügbar unter https://fcc.report/FCC-ID/VNP-AL/4296618.pdf, zuletzt geprüft am 03.05.2024

MED-EL (2022b): RONDO 3 Audioprozessor. Produktkatalog. Online verfügbar unter https://www.medel.com/de/hearing-solutions/accessories/product-catalogue, zuletzt geprüft am 25.02.2022

MED-EL (2022c): SONNET 2 Audioprozessor. Produktkatalog. Online verfügbar unter https://www.medel.com/de/hearing-solutions/accessories/product-catalogue, zuletzt geprüft am 25.02.2022

Merse, S. (2020): Übersetzungsprozesse in der Arzt-Patienten-Kommunikation. In: Gillessen, A., Golsabahi-Broclawski, S., Biakowski, A. und Broclawski, A. (Hrsg.): Interkulturelle Kommunikation in der Medizin, S. 61–71, Berlin, Heidelberg, Springer

Montano, J. J.; Spitzer, J. B. (2021): Adult Audiologic Rehabilitation. Third Edition. San Diego, Plural Publishing Inc.

Oticon Medical (2018): Neuro 2. Bedienungsanleitung. Online verfügbar unter https://www.manualslib.de/manual/403151/Oticon-Medical-Neuro-2.html, zuletzt geprüft am 25.02.2022.

Oticon Medical (2022): Bleiben Sie verbunden. Online verfügbar unter https://www.oticonmedical.com/de/cochlear-implants/solutions/connectivity. Zugegriffen: 25.02.2022.

Rötz, W.; Eichler, T.; Sudhoff, H.; Todt, I. (2022): Überwindung der Sprachbarriere in der Hör-Sprachrehabilitation mittels multilingualer Konversationsapplikationen. [unpublished source]

Scharff Rethfeldt, W. (2017): Evidenzen zu Empfehlungen und Ansätzen in der Sprachtherapie mit mehrsprachigen Kindern. In: Forum Logopädie 6 (31), S. 18–23

Schwemmle, C. (2012): Hörverarbeitung, Gehirnplastizität und Hörtherapie. In: Sprache Stimme Gehör 36 (04), e81–e85. https://doi.org/10.1055/s-0032-1327633

Statistisches Bundesamt (2021): Bevölkerung, Migration und Integration. Online verfügbar unter https://www.destatis.de/DE/Themen/Gesellschaft-Umwelt/Bevoelkerung/Migration-Integration/_inhalt.html, zuletzt geprüft am 13.10.2021

Tremblay, K. (2007): Training-Related Changes in the Brain: Evidence from Human Auditory-Evoked Potentials. In: Semin Hear 28 (2), S. 120–132. https://doi.org/10.1055/s-2007-973438

Weltgesundheitsorganisation (WHO) (2005): Internationale Klassifikation der Funktionsfähigkeit, behinderung und gesundheit (ICF). Hg. V. Deutsches Institut für Medizinische Dokumentation und Information (DIMDI).

Zeh, R. & Baumann, U. (2015). Stationäre Rehabilitationsmaßnahmen bei erwachsenen CI-Trägern. Ergebnisse in Abhängigkeit von der Dauer der Taubheit, Nutzungsdauer und Alter. In: HNO 63 (8), S. 557–576. https://doi.org/10.1007/s00106-015-0037-2

Preparation of the Therapy

4.1 Coordination Between Surgery, Audiology, and Therapy

The supplying process with a CI requires extensive exchange between various specialist areas in order to provide the patient with the best possible conditions and the success of the provision. This affects all topics from the indication, through the surgical intervention, the technical fitting, to the therapeutic treatment in the form of auditory training.

4.1.1 Coordination Between Audiology and Surgery

Once the patient has decided on a manufacturer, the surgeon must choose a suitable implant and exchange information with the CI technician about the order of the implant and the sound processor **before the implantation**.

During the surgical intervention, the CI technician receives information from the surgeon about the course of the implantation, such as the found condition of the cochlea and the details about the insertion (e.g., access to the cochlea, insertion depth, number of inserted electrodes).

Subsequently, the function of the implant is checked by the CI technician using the individual manufacturer's software. Normally, there is a complete insertion of all electrodes into the scala tympani, with complete functionality of the implant. For the exceptions, a careful check for any defects on the electrodes is necessary to find out whether an exchange of the implant or the switching off of individual electrodes must take place. The software also tests the auditory nerve's reactions to electrical stimulation by the electrodes, i.e., over a wide frequency range, for the first time. Among other things, these measurements are important parameters for the subsequent fitting of the sound processor (Basta 2009).

© The Author(s), under exclusive license to Springer-Verlag GmbH, DE, part of Springer Nature 2025
W. Rötz, B. Bertram, *Cochlear Implantation in Adults*,
https://doi.org/10.1007/978-3-662-72230-5_4

After the implantation and a several-week-long healing phase, the fitting process of the sound processor begins. About the course, especially abnormalities (e.g., co-stimulation of the facial nerve, newly occurring balance problems, or a missing benefit in the hearing test), the CI technician informs the surgeon. In this way, possible connections to the medical history and surgery can be established, and suitable treatment solutions can be found.

4.1.2 Coordination Between Surgery and Therapy

The possibility of exchange between the surgeon and the therapist is strongly dependent on the structures of the clinic. While here mutual feedback is at least conceivable, an exchange between the surgeon and therapists in independent practices is extremely rare. The main contact with the therapist is through the audiological department staff.

In the context of an exchange, the surgeon can inform the therapist about special features during the surgical intervention and thus about possible challenges in auditory training. About the individual course of therapy, the therapist can then provide feedback to the surgeon.

4.1.3 Coordination Between Audiology and Therapy

After the initial fitting of the sound processor, auditory training begins. The CI technician and the therapist should be in as close contact as possible and exchange information about the development of speech understanding with the CI. The therapist must be informed about aspects of the fitting in order to be able to address them in the therapy. Likewise, the CI technician relies on the feedback from the therapist in order to make the fitting of the sound processor as precise as possible. Since these are very detailed results from the therapy, they are described in detail in Sect. 5.3.

In mutual exchange, the following aspects should be considered:

- Information from the exchange with the surgeon
- Deactivated electrodes
- Unwanted co-stimulation of the facial nerve while the auditory nerve is stimulated by the implant
- Hardware and software problems
- Fitting details (programs, volume, etc.)
- Wearing times of the sound processor
- Ordered additional technical accessories
- Implementation of feedback from therapy
- Requirements for the therapist, e.g., functions that should be tried out in auditory training

More information on individual fitting options can be found in Sect. 1.7.

4.2 Anamnesis Based on the International Classification of Functioning, Disability and Health (ICF)

An anamnesis interview is always tailored to the reason for therapy. Since hearing impairment affects various areas of patients' lives, the therapist collects additional aspects such as limits and resources in the professional and private environment. The components of the ICF provide a suitable basis for designing an anamnesis form.

4.2.1 Body Functions and Structures

CI users have an impairment in the hearing process and sometimes also damage to the balance function. In this regard, the exact circumstances of the cause and the course are evaluated. Both ears should always be considered, even if only one side is supplied with a CI.

Other diseases not related to the ear and their medical treatment can also influence the course of therapy. These are mainly cognitive impairments and medications that disrupt cognition.

> **Questions in the Anamnesis About Diseases and the Course of Hearing Impairment**
> - Cause of hearing impairment
> - Onset of hearing impairment
> - Changes in hearing impairment over time
> - Time of deafness
> - Past ear surgeries
> - Abnormalities during the operation (implantation of the CI)
> - Further impairments of the ear (balance disorders and tinnitus)
> - Comorbidities and medications

If a patient is already **prelingually** (before completion of language acquisition) **hard of hearing** or **deaf**, certain frequencies may never have been perceived. This can affect both the patient's pronunciation and the habituation to the sound of certain speech sounds, as well as their tolerance to higher volumes. Sometimes, patients only notice with a CI that their own pronunciation is conspicuous and wish to improve it on their own initiative. In the first weeks and months after the initial fitting, pronunciation often changes by itself due to improved auditory feedback (acoustic review of one's own spoken language), and at this point, if desired, information about the possibilities of articulation therapy can also be provided.

If the **hearing loss or deafness** only occurred **postlingually** (after completion of language acquisition), the timing is particularly relevant for auditory training. In connection with the patient's age, this results in the duration of the hearing disorder. The longer a deafness or untreated hearing loss existed, the more difficult it is to predict the duration and the success of therapy (Sect. 1.2).

A **unilateral deafness with normal hearing on the opposite side (SSD)** mainly has consequences in the temporary masking of the opposite ear for training reasons. An advantage for patients is that they always have the possibility of comparison with the normal hearing ear. This sometimes facilitates habituation to the hearing impressions with the CI. At the same time, especially in the case of sudden deafness, it can lead to frustration when patients only realize at this point how much hearing with a CI differs from the healthy ear. It takes a lot of empathy from the therapist and patience from the patient to accompany and endure the learning process with the CI. It is certain that the acoustic perception will change over time and will generally improve both objectively and subjectively.

4.2.2 Environmental Factors

In addition to the "body functions and structures", the domain "Products and Technology" of the "Environmental Factors" is considered, which deals with the **individual care of hearing loss or deafness**. The better an ear was supplied before an implantation of a CI, the more promising the prognosis with the CI. Each CI manufacturer has its own sound processors and additional technical accessories. In exchange with the CI technicians and when using **additional technical accessories** in therapy, the individual's care must be known. In addition, the use of other devices should be asked to possibly use them in therapy or to advise patients on procurement.

Furthermore, within the framework of domains three ("Support and Relationships") and four ("Attitudes") of the ICF, it should be asked how the patient perceives the **support and acceptance of his hearing impairment by others**. Both close family members and friends, as well as other people with whom the patient interacts in his everyday life, contribute essentially to the patient's acceptance of disability with their care and attitude towards the special needs. If patients experience the topic of hearing impairment as a taboo or a weakness in their environment, they may already be hindered on the way to acceptance. This promotes self-doubt and a withdrawal from social interaction, which affects the category "Activity and Participation" of the ICF. For auditory training, this can specifically mean that independent training at home is difficult, and the willingness to test additional technical accessories in everyday life is low in order to hide the hearing impairment.

> **Questions in the Anamnesis Interview About Environmental Factors**
> - Type of hearing system (both sides)
> - Change in the supply of hearing systems over time
> - For CI: manufacturer, sound processor, additional technical accessories, compatibility with the hearing system of the opposite ear
> - Supplying facilities, possibly with address and phone number (hearing aid acoustician or CI-supplying clinic)
> - Further additional technical accessories and their use in everyday life (Sect. 4.4)
> - Consideration and support in the private environment
> - Consideration and support in the professional environment

4.2.3 Activity and Participation

Impaired hearing requires an increased level of concentration and attention when communicating. This usually leads to faster exhaustion and fatigue than for people with normal hearing. As people with a hearing impairment operate in an environment created by hearing people, this often leads to **expectations** that the hearing-impaired person cannot fulfil or cannot fully fulfil. Especially for people who become hard of hearing or deaf later in life, it can be a challenge to accept the new reality of life. Patients must therefore learn to reassess their **ability to participate** in life and how to deal with it. In order to optimize the framework conditions as much as possible, the first step is to improve speech comprehension in everyday communication and the sensible use of **additional technical communication-supporting accessories** in everyday life. This benefits the patient in "Listening," "Focusing Attention," "Dealing with Stress and Psychological Demands," "Communicating as a Receiver or Sender," and various "Interpersonal Interactions and Relationships" of the category "Activity and Participation" in the ICF. At the same time, it is not only important to constantly redefine one's own limits, but also to recognize **relaxing and empowering resources** and integrate them into everyday life.

> **Questions in the Anamnesis Interview About Activity and Participation**
> - Expectations of one's own performance (private and professional)
> - Measures to support communication in everyday situations
> - Contact with fellow sufferers and counseling centers
> - Measures for relaxation and integration of hearing breaks into everyday life
> - Hobbies

4.2.4 Personal Factors

Due to the high individuality, the "personal factors" in the ICF were not classified in more detail. However, there is some anamnestic relevant information that can be assigned to this area.

The **age of the patient** plays an important role in connection with the time at which the hearing loss or deafness occurred. It can also be revealing to find out at what time the patient grew up. World events and societal norms often influenced the type of medical care people received and how disabilities were handled. For example, indications for hearing systems have changed over the decades, or certain provisions, such as the CI, were only invented. During times of war and postwar periods, or during refugee movements, medical care was sometimes severely limited, so that patients themselves had little knowledge about the course and causes of their own hearing loss. This can distort a prognosis for hearing success with the CI.

In connection with the questions about "environmental factors" and "activity and participation," it is important to ask about the **current professional activity**. The **native language** also plays a role in the implementation of auditory training. If it doesn't match the therapist's native language, they must consider how the therapy can be structured (Sect. 3.3.4). The patient's native language can also be sign language. However, this is very rare, as the prospect of success in understanding spoken language is low in cases of prelingual deafness. It is more likely that prelingually severely hearing-impaired people are competent in sign language as well as having spoken language skills. Above all, the choice of materials in therapy is then strongly determined by the extent of the patient's verbal language competencies. Each sign language is a standalone and recognized language with its own grammatical system. Therefore, the grammar of verbal spoken language can be challenging at the sentence or text level. In addition, sign languages are less metaphorical, which is why, for example, proverbs and idioms of verbal spoken language are rather less known. The therapy material is therefore adapted to the patient's knowledge.

A special case is **illiteracy or limited reading and writing skills**. Since illiteracy is a very sensitive topic, it should be carefully considered whether and at what point the reading and writing skills are required. With appropriate education and professional activity, it can generally be assumed that patients can read and write. If patients with limited reading and writing skills need visual support in exercises, the therapist must have a repertoire of visual aids and exercises.

Also, to be assigned to the "personal factors" is the **motivation and goal setting** of the patient (Sect. 4.4) and his individual resilience, which has a great influence on his patience, the perseverance in therapy, and on dealing with his own hearing loss. This is not explicitly asked, but can often be better assessed through a detailed anamnesis interview and makes it easier for the therapist to find a balanced measure between emotional accompaniment and performance demand (Cf. World Health Organization (WHO) 2005).

> **Personal History Questions**
> - Date of birth (age)
> - Education and profession
> - Native language
> - Other languages
> - Literacy
> - Objectives

4.3 Diagnostics and Findings

After the anamnesis interview, diagnostics follow to find out how the patient perceives auditory impressions (Heinemann 2014, p. 24). This is difficult in the case of CI patients, as there is no standardized diagnostic material for use in auditory training. Nevertheless, to determine an appropriate starting level of exercise difficulty, one can rely on the evaluation of the audiological diagnostics with the CI and on various possibilities of non-standardized examination procedures in auditory training. This may provide insights into understanding with the CI, which do not always correspond to observations in later training. Therefore, the findings are always interpreted in conjunction with factors such as cognitive and linguistic abilities, or the type and duration of provision of hearing systems. Since the exercises in auditory training are very variable and easily changeable, the level can be adjusted without complications.

4.3.1 Speech Therapy Diagnostics and Findings

In the absence of suitable diagnostic material for auditory training, the therapist can only compare the patient with other patients using the evaluation of the audiological diagnostics. Nevertheless, there are various possibilities to at least represent the progress of the individual patient. This means that the chosen test procedures must be repeated at larger intervals in order to obtain a reliable finding.

Vowel and Consonant Identification
The assignment of individual sounds only allows minor conclusions about a general understanding of spoken language. However, one can gain an impression of how the patient perceives certain frequency ranges.

Zeh and Baumann (2015) describe the procedure for eight vowels and as well as 20 consonants related to the German language. These are spoken a maximum of twice, without the patient seeing the mouth shape, and the patient repeats them. Subsequently, the percentage of correctly repeated sounds is calculated.

If you want to shorten the duration of the procedure, you can reduce the number of speech sounds. It is important to test sounds from all frequency ranges. For this purpose, the six so-called Ling sounds /m, u, i, a, sh, s/ could be used. They are normally used in diagnostics with children with hearing impairments and cover the entire language area (Ling 1976).

Speech Tracking
Another common test is the speech-tracking test to check language comprehension at the text level. For the procedure, a text is needed, which is read to the patient in phrases. Each read phrase is repeated by the patient. The number of repeated words within a minute is determined. Zeh and Baumann (2015) describe the procedure with and without a mouth shape to gain additional information about the extent to which the patient uses visual information for understanding.

However, if the test is repeated after some time, there is a risk that the patient will remember the content and thus falsify the test result. If you read the text further or use a new one, the results are also limited in comparability. The texts would likely vary in their number of words of certain lengths. There might also be differences in the level of content difficulty. Counting syllables instead of words could be a solution. The syllable is considered a basic unit for determining speech speed (Uhmann 1997, p. 190) and is also used in other areas of speech and language therapy, such as in the diagnosis of stuttering. However, switching to syllables alone would not eliminate all inaccuracies, as, for example, the number of written syllables differs from the number of spoken ones (Uhmann 1997, p. 191).

4.3.2 Audiological Diagnosis and Findings

Even before the implantation, various audiological diagnostic procedures are carried out to determine the CI-indication. Among other things, a pure tone and speech audiogram are carried out with and without a hearing system (Todt 2009). These subjective hearing tests are also carried out after the implantation. This makes the benefit of the CI visible, both in comparison with the condition before the implantation and with the results of other patients.

For the therapist, the results can serve to determine the starting level of the exercises. For this, the therapist needs a current hearing test (standard in Germany: aided threshold with CI, single and multi-syllable test in the free field with CI) or the written evaluation of it. To obtain a finding to determine the starting level, the therapist looks at the tests in context. The test results can be transmitted via contact with the CI technicians or the patient directly.

▶ **Tip** Different clinics have different audiometers and versions of test software. This influences the symbols that represent the individual values in the hearing test. If the symbols cannot be clearly assigned to a test, a legend of the symbols or a written evaluation can be requested in the clinic.

4.3 Diagnostics and Findings

The following classification of the results is only a suggestion for therapy. In individual cases, a decision must be made in conjunction with the patient's prerequisites.

4.3.2.1 Categorization of Test Results
Aided Threshold with CI (Pure-Tone Audiogram)
The aided threshold can be used to determine whether speech can be perceived at all and thus provides a first orientation.

Ideally, all frequencies are perceived at a similar volume, i.e., a threshold whose measurement points all lie in a small area on the Y-axis (speech level in dB) in the pure-tone audiogram. If the threshold is difficult to classify at first glance, the Pure-Tone Average (PTA-4) can be calculated and used for categorization. For this, the average value of the frequencies 0.5 kHz, 1 kHz, 2 kHz, and 4 kHz is determined.

- **Good**: -10 dB to 30 dB: The patient has good prerequisites for the perception of speech.
- **Uncertain**: > 31 dB: It is uncertain which parts of speech the patient perceives how. The higher the levels to which the threshold is shifted, the more difficult it is to understand.

Multisyllabic Test (Speech Audiogram)
A test of the Freiburg Speech Comprehension Test is the Freiburg Number Test. This consists of multi-syllable numbers, which CI patients, due to the limited number of possible numbers and the respective word length, often understand very well early on. The division into two categories is therefore sufficient to make a rough estimate.

- **Good:** ≥ 50 dB
- **Uncertain:** < 50 dB

Monosyllabic Test (Speech Audiogram)
In addition to the multisyllables, there is the Freiburg Monosyllabic Test, which consists of fixed groups of monosyllables. Monosyllables are very demanding due to their brevity and are therefore often only well understood in the course of fittings and training sessions. The understanding of monosyllables is rated at 65 dB.

- **Low monosyllabic understanding:** 0–15%
- **Medium monosyllabic understanding:** >15–50%
- **Good monosyllabic understanding:** >50–100%

4.3.2.2 Determine Starting Level

When the individual categories are combined, the starting level for the beginning of therapy can be derived from this. In this book, difficulty levels 1–4 have been established, with level 1 corresponding to very easy exercises and level 4 to difficult exercises.

The following combinations are most likely:

- **Aided threshold uncertain, multisyllables uncertain, monosyllables low:** very easy starting level (single sounds—difficulty level 1)
- **Aided threshold good, multisyllables uncertain, monosyllables low:** very easy to easy starting level (single sounds or words—difficulty level 1)
- **Aided threshold good, multisyllables good, monosyllables medium:** medium starting level (words—difficulty level 2)
- **Aided threshold good, multisyllables good, monosyllables good:** high starting level (sentences—difficulty level 1)

Other combinations are very unlikely. Possibly one of the tests was not performed correctly (e.g., test instruction imprecise) or the patient gave incorrect information (was, for example, unfocused or very tense). However, therapy can still be started according to the suggested procedure in Chap. 5.

4.4 Goals Based on the ICF

The objectives of audio therapy and auditory training often overlap. Each therapist must decide for themself, depending on their training and experience, to what extent they can offer support from both areas to the individual patient.

At the beginning of therapy, patients often ask why they need therapy with their CI from a speech and language therapist; after all, they have no problem with speaking. At the same time, they almost invariably express the desire for better hearing when asked about their goal with the CI. This answer seems obvious at first, but is very unspecific. The task of the therapist is therefore to educate about the possibilities and limits of therapy, as well as to work with the patient to specify his desire for improved hearing to convert into a realistic goal of will (Eberspächer 2009). The patient must be willing to bring about a change and make the necessary efforts. The goals should always be realistic and concrete in order to make the achievement verifiable (Mayer et al. 2003).

First, the question arises as to what the desire "to hear better" means for patients in concrete terms. As a rule, this means an increased participation in communication through better understanding. This implies that the mere optimization of the sound processor fitting is not sufficient, but only forms the basis for the actual purpose of the therapy (Diller 2009). For goal setting, further individual factors of the patient must be included (Braun 2016), for which the anamnestic findings can be used. By dividing the therapy into basic and follow-up therapy as well as long-term follow-up

4.4 Goals Based on the ICF

care, the current guideline also recommends such an approach (DGHNO-KHC e.V. 2020). Oriented on the categories of the ICF, areas for goal formulation can be determined.

4.4.1 Body Functions and Structures

At the beginning of therapy, the "function of hearing" should be restored as best as possible. This corresponds to the goal formulated in the guidelines of optimizing the sound processor fitting in the context of basic therapy. The basis for this is the interlocking of the sound processor fitting and auditory training (Diller 2009; Illg 2017). Individual goals in this phase of therapy are primarily based on the prerequisites and the willingness to cooperate or motivation of the patient (Dahm 1998, p. 123; Diller 2009).

> **Areas for Goal Formulation**
> - Volume setting
> - Frequency perception
> - Hearing and understanding verbal spoken language (initially only through repetition)
> - Independent training at home

4.4.2 Environmental Factors

The "products and technologies" named in the category of "environmental factors" are daily companions of the patient from the time of implantation. Since the correct use of the technical devices (sound processor and additional technical accessories) forms the basis for reliable communication, the patient should know and be able to use the technology. Patients should know at least the most basic care and maintenance tasks. In addition, patients should be familiar with important functions (e.g., switching on and off, volume control, and, if possible, changing programs) and be able to perform them independently.

In the context of the domains "Support and Relationship" and "Attitudes," other people can be involved in the therapy, or the patient can be enabled to express and communicate their needs.

> **Areas for Goal Formulation**
> - Handling of the sound processor and the additional technical accessories
> - Assessment of the course and success of therapy
> - Education of the environment
> - Communication of needs

4.4.3 Activity and Participation

The category of "activity and participation" contains aspects that are assigned in the guidelines for follow-up therapy and long-term follow-up care (DGHNO-KHC e.V. 2020, pp. 12–13). After successful sound processor optimization, understanding is elevated to a communicative level to increase interaction with others. Possible limitations in participation should also be recognized and addressed. Together, the use of additional technical accessories is tested and measures to relieve concentration in everyday life are discussed.

> **Areas for Goal Formulation**
> - Understanding verbal spoken language up to a complex communication level
> - Use of additional technical accessories in everyday situations
> - Limits of CI use
> - Recognizing and utilizing resources

4.4.4 Personal Factors

Especially after sudden hearing loss, the new hearing situation may require patients to redefine private and professional goals and to question their own habits or attitudes. The patients have to deal with established aspects of their personality. This often causes many doubts, questions, and sometimes feelings of mourning. In the processing process, this ultimately means new perspectives and paths that can be taken (cf. World Health Organization (WHO) 2005).

> **Area for Goal Formulation**
> - Acceptance of disability

Literature

Basta, D. (2009): Perioperatives Monitoring objektiv-audiologischer Daten im Rahmen der Cochlear-Implant-Versorgung. In: Ernst, Battmer, Todt (2009): Cochlear Implant heute, S. 31–38, Springer

Braun, Astrid (2016): Cochlea-Implantat (CI)-Rehabilitation bei postlingual ertaubten CI-Trägern. In: *Hörakustik* (9), S. 50–52

Dahm, M. C. (1998): Indikation, Kontraindikation und Voruntersuchung bei Erwachsenen. In: Thomas Lenarz (Hg.): Cochlea-Implantat. Ein praktischer Leitfaden für die Versorgung von Kindern und Erwachsenen. Berlin: Springer, S. 122–135

DGHNO-KHC e.V. (2020): S2K-Leitlinie. Cochlea-Implantat Versorgung: AWMF-Register (017/071)

Diller, G. (2009): (Re)habilitation nach Versorgung mit einem Kochleaimplantat. In: *HNO* 57 (7), S. 649–656. https://doi.org/10.1007/s00106-009-1922-3

Eberspächer, H. (2009): Ressource Ich. Stressmanagement in Beruf und Alltag. 3., erw. Aufl. München: Hanser (Erfolg + Karriere)

Heinemann, S. (2014): Der Weg zum neuen Hören. Aspekte der Beratung und Therapie von erwachsenen Cochlea-Implantat-Trägern. In: *Spektrum Patholinguistik* (7), S. 13–39

Illg, A. (2017): Rehabilitation bei Kindern und Erwachsenen: Ein Überblick. In: *HNO* 65 (7), S. 552–560. https://doi.org/10.1007/s00106-016-0311-y

Ling, D. (1976): Speech and the hearing-impaired child. Theory and practice. Washington: Alexander Graham Bell Association for the Deaf

Mayer, J.; Görlich, P.; Eberspächer, H. (2003): Mentales Gehtraining. Berlin, Heidelberg: Springer Berlin Heidelberg

Todt, I. (2009): Cochlear-Implant-Voruntersuchungen. In: Ernst, Battmer, Todt (2009): Cochlear Implant heute S. 27–30. Berlin, Heidelberg: Springer Berlin Heidelberg

Uhmann, S. (Hg.) (1997): Grammatische Regeln und konversationelle Strategien: DE GRUYTER

Weltgesundheitsorganisation (WHO) (2005): Internationale Klassifikation der Funktionsfähigkeit, Behinderung und Gesundheit (ICF). Hg. v. Deutsches Institut für Medizinische Dokumentation und Information (DIMDI)

Zeh, R. (2015) igkeit von der Dauer der Taubheit, Nutzungsdauer und Alter. In: *HNO* 63 (8), S. 557–576. https://doi.org/10.1007/s00106-015-0037-2

Structure and Contents of Therapy

Auditory training with adult CI users aims to match existing auditory impressions with the new perception provided by the CI. In this process, various levels are passed through, which show parallels to child hearing development and are closely interlinked with language development. While hearing development in children takes place for the first time, postlingually deafened patients go through this process repeatedly. Since they already have hearing experience, learning to hear with the CI happens much faster. Norman P. Erber (1982) describes the hierarchical structure of these achievements in his book on auditory training (*Auditory Training*) with hearing-impaired children. First, the presence of acoustic impressions is registered (*Detection*), then differences in the acoustic signals are recognized (*Discrimination*, often also called differentiation), before they can be assigned (*Identification*). The highest requirement is the *Understanding* of the content.

Each exercise area in auditory training with adults can serve several levels of this process.

Levels of Hearing Development According to Erber
- Detection
- Discrimination
- Identification
- Understanding

5.1 Exercise Areas and Their Implementation

The necessity of practicing in various nonlinguistic and linguistic areas is widely agreed upon in the literature. The areas of noise, speech sounds, words, sentences, texts, and understanding on the phone are repeatedly mentioned (Heinemann 2014; Diller 2009; Lenarz 1998, p. 137; Illg 2017). In addition, for example, understanding background noise (Diller 2009; Heinemann 2014), the use of electronic media or sound carriers (Diller 2009; Illg 2017), or instruments and music, as well as spatial hearing (Diller 2009), are discussed. In a study, Anton and Otero (2018, p. 57) surveyed speech therapists on the content of the actual postoperative therapy with CI patients. The surveys revealed that the exercise areas of speech sounds and noises, words, sentences, and texts, as well as exercises in background noise, receive the most attention. However, not only is the selection of the exercise area important, but also its implementation.

The areas of detection and discrimination take up a lot of space in many descriptions of content in auditory training. Following a hierarchical approach, Lenarz (1998, pp. 137f.) described the implementation of exercises for noise perception and differentiation, followed by exercises for the perception and distinction of speech sounds in syllables. These exercises are intended to help the patient learn to listen again and consciously perceive noises. However, current literature also points to the need to regularly incorporate detection and discrimination into the therapy process. Before exercises for word understanding take place, Diller (2009) also first mentions the therapy contents, noise detection and discrimination, vowel and consonant discrimination, and additionally exercises for recognizing rhythmic-prosodic language structures. Braun (2016, p. 50) also recommends noise and sound work as a preliminary exercise at the beginning of therapy. This approach is still pursued in current therapeutic practice (Anton and Otero 2018).

The best possible understanding of spoken language in various situations can be seen as the main concern of a CI supply. Ideally, this means as few restrictions as possible in everyday communication. Diller (1997, p. 91) describes this as an open understanding of verbal spoken language. However, in auditory training, several sessions are often used for detection and discrimination exercises and the recognition of prosodic-rhythmic structures, instead of for identification and understanding. Especially, the integration of this into the process of real communication, which is so relevant to everyday life, often receives too little attention or only takes place at a late stage in auditory training.

The rapid technical development of recent years and the expansion of the indication criteria have led to ever better sound results when listening with the CI, which is why the weighting of the exercise areas and their implementation in auditory training should be questioned and restructured.

5.1.1 Systematics of the Exercise Areas

Possible exercise areas can be divided into linguistic and nonlinguistic sub-areas.

1. In the *nonlinguistic areas*, exercises for detection, discrimination, and identification can be carried out. This affects the exercise areas of noises, tones, melody and music, voices, and spatial hearing.
2. The *linguistic areas* of speech sounds, syllables, words, phrases, sentences, texts, and everyday communication serve all levels, including understanding, although the area of individual speech sounds has a clearly subordinate function in this. *Further linguistic areas* include making phone calls and listening and understanding in noise. Although they are also based on language, all linguistic exercise areas are run through within these two areas according to the sequence shown.

The increase in linguistic exercise areas is achieved by approximating the utterances (items) in their complexity (length and content) to everyday communication. The nonlinguistic areas can be variably integrated into the therapy according to the exercise goal.

> **Nonlinguistic and Linguistic Exercise Areas**
> Nonlinguistic exercise areas
>
> - Noises
> - Tones
> - Melody and music
> - Voices
> - Spatial hearing
>
> Linguistic exercise areas with increasing approximation to everyday communication
>
> - Speech sounds
> - Syllables
> - Words
> - Phrases
> - Sentences
> - Texts
> - Everyday communication
>
> Further linguistic exercise areas
>
> - Making phone calls
> - Understanding in noise

Within the areas, there is a need for additional weighting according to the individual difficulty level of each exercise. The difficulty of the exercise depends on various linguistic parameters, the presentation of the exercise, and the connection with the cognitive demands of communication.

5.1.1.1 Linguistic Parameters
Item Length
The more reduced the acoustic information is, the more difficult it is to understand. This leads, for example, to the fact that monosyllabic words are more challenging than polysyllables.

Frequency
The rarer the use in everyday language, the more difficult it is to compare with already existing auditory impressions.

Frequency Variability of Speech Sounds
An utterance that offers hardly any prosodic clues due to minor changes in pitch becomes very blurred in sound and is difficult to understand.

Word Class
The more tangible the content of a word is, the easier it is to understand. Content words (e.g., nouns and verbs) are therefore easier to understand than function words (e.g., articles and prepositions).

Phonological Similarity in Comparative Exercises
The more phonologically similar the items are, the more difficult they are to differentiate from each other. Minimal pairs will therefore be more difficult to distinguish than two words that differ greatly in sound.

Association Strength in the Exercise Context
If an exercise is given a semantic frame, also called a closed set, items that correspond more to this are easier to understand than items that correspond less to the content context (cf. Heinemann 2014, p. 25)

5.1.1.2 Connection with Cognitive Demands in Communication
Communication consists of more aspects than just the pure verbal exchange, such as nonverbal information exchange. This part of communication is deliberately omitted here, as auditory training primarily deals with the verbal aspect of communication.

How well a patient can understand acoustically with his CI allows conclusions to be drawn about the functionality of the individual fitting of the sound processor. For this, only the principle of "speaking (by the therapist) and repeating (by the patient)" is necessary in auditory training. However, this only forms the basis for the ability to conduct a verbal conversation. Communication goes beyond this level and requires additional performance from the patient. This includes understanding the information in terms of content, recognizing the speaker's intention, planning a reaction, responding, and remembering what was heard throughout the entire process (cf. Beyer and Gerlach 2011, p. 30).

> **Cognitive Performance in Communication**
> 1. Remembering what was heard throughout the entire communication process (Memory)
> 2. Understanding content (Meaning)
> 3. Recognizing the speaker's intention (Interpretation)
> 4. Planning a reaction (Processing)
> 5. Responding or engaging with what was said (Reaction)

The more complex the exercise is in terms of additional cognitive requirements, the more concentration and attention will be demanded of the patient. Therefore, the integration of aspects that go beyond acoustic understanding should only take place when "speaking and repeating" no longer requires the patient's full concentration and attention.

Fear of Dementia
Patients often worryingly mention the suspicion of possibly developing dementia over time, as they notice an increasing forgetfulness in everyday life. This existential concern is associated with great fears and must always be taken seriously. Although a therapist in auditory training does not have the competence of a medical assessment about the actual cause, the frequent forgetting is usually explainable by a limited capacity for intake. The challenge of acoustic understanding is sometimes so immense that there simply isn't the capacity for additional cognitive performances. This not only leads to forgetfulness but also to increased fatigue. In case of doubt, a neurological clarification should always be carried out by the responsible medical staff.

5.1.1.3 Presentation of Exercise Material
By linking auditory with visual information, the patient can be gradually introduced to higher levels of difficulty. The exclusively acoustic presentation represents the highest goal. If the patient needs a lot of visual assistance during an exercise, this can be frustrating. At this point, it may be helpful to supplement the exercise from the outset with a permanent visual assistance. The target item is always presented acoustically, while the visual part varies. This involves the presentation of items in written or pictorial form.

▶ The visual presentation of an item often leads to patients only pointing to the heard item, instead of repeating it. In order to achieve as many repetitions of an item as possible and to give the patient the opportunity to compare acoustically again and again, he can be asked to repeat the items instead of pointing to them.

Visual (Writing or Picture)
The spoken word is presented in written or pictorial form during the acoustic presentation, or a selection of written images or illustrations is given.

Mixed: Acoustic and Visual
The patient hears an item while one part of the item is presented visually in the form of a picture or text.

Acoustic
The patient hears an item, but receives no visual information.

> **Tip** If a pictorial selection is given in the exercise, all items should be named once to ensure that the patient understands which picture is associated with which item. Since pictures have a certain room for interpretation, it can also happen that the patient has a different item in mind than what is acoustically presented. This makes the comparison with stored acoustic impressions difficult or sometimes impossible.
>
> Nevertheless, the pictorial representation is generally somewhat more difficult than the written one. The patient must remember the exact assignment of the verbal spoken language to the picture throughout the entire exercise, while writing is always clear. The more unspecific the illustration is, the higher the additional memory performance.

If all possibilities for classifying the difficulty of an exercise are taken into account, this ultimately leads to an exercise sequence in which the exercises of one level of difficulty from one area always follow the same level of difficulty of an exercise area with a shorter length of utterance. The respective level of difficulty for the exercises in Chap. 6 is always noted under "Level of Difficulty."

The starting point for the exercise sequence is the initially determined starting level through the diagnostic results (Sect. 4.3). Since the starting level is not always clear at the beginning and therefore requires a flexible approach, it can happen that within a therapy session several areas or also levels of difficulty are passed through.

Exercise Sequence at Starting Level Words—Difficulty Level 1

Words—Difficulty level 1
  Phrases—Difficulty level 1
  Sentences—Difficulty level 1
  Texts—Difficulty level 1
  Speech sounds—Difficulty level 2
  Syllables—Difficulty level 2
  Words—Difficulty Level 2
  etc. ◄

This approach serves as a guide. A deviation such as skipping exercises or returning to a previous difficulty level is always possible and may be necessary for some patients due to daily form, a recent fitting of the sound processor, or special prerequisites due to the anamnesis. For example, if a diagnosed dementia or aphasia is present, it may happen that higher difficulty levels cannot be reached. The more complex the exercises are in content, the more difficult it can be for such patients to deliver the required performance or for the therapists to distinguish hearing and understanding errors from symptoms of other diseases.

The biggest challenge is to find a seamless transition between the difficulty levels so that the patient remains equally challenged as the requirements increase. This is not always successful and sometimes leads to a higher effort or error rate.

▶ If difficulty increases are not explicitly mentioned, patients often do not notice them and therefore perceive an increased effort or error rate as a deterioration. At this point, the patient should be reassured that this is due to the increased difficulty and thus represents progress in auditory training.

The focus on the understanding performance constantly demanded in auditory training can put patients under pressure. Accordingly, the disappointment is sometimes huge when the feeling arises that they cannot always meet this requirement. A proven way to reduce this pressure is to divert the patient's concentration to another action (e.g., a game action). This often does not make things more difficult, but rather relaxing, and subsequently leads to a more relaxed listening and improved speech reception function. Appropriate suggestions for adult-friendly games can be found in the exercise overview.

▶ **Tip** Instructions for the following areas can be found in the exercises for speech and hearing therapy in Chap. 6.
- Speech sounds
- Syllables
- Words
- Phrases
- Sentences
- Texts
- Noises
- Tones
- Melody and music
- Voices

5.1.2 Basic Rules of Exercise Execution

Without adherence to some important basic rules, an assessment of the understanding performance with the CI is hardly possible. This in turn has a major influence on the feedback regarding the fitting of the sound processor and ultimately also on the progress of the individual patient.

5.1.2.1 Beginning of Therapy

The intensity or volume is slowly increased to a higher level in the fittings, so the auditory impressions after the first fittings are sometimes too quiet to cover part of the speech range. Also, the first hearing test with CI is not performed directly after the initial fitting in many clinics, so the diagnostic indications for assessing a starting level in auditory training are insufficient. Therefore, auditory training should only start after about two to three adjustments and after a hearing test has been conducted. Otherwise, the training could lead to unnecessary frustration for the patient. Since the procedure varies from clinic to clinic, this information is asked of the patient or directly in the clinic.

5.1.2.2 Temporary Masking of the Opposite Ear

Until an initially optimal fitting of the sound processor has been found for the patient, practice must first be done without the help of the other ear (Heinemann 2014, p. 23; Braun 2016, p. 51). The brain always evaluates all available acoustic information from both ears. A conscious ignoring of one ear is not possible and is therefore artificially induced. Since the correct masking affects the entire therapy process, it must be carried out particularly conscientiously. Depending on the hearing status, a hearing threshold or an aided threshold can be helpful, but do not mandatorily have to be available.

▶ **Aided Threshold** An aided threshold is a hearing threshold with hearing systems. The measurement is done in the sound field, i.e., via speakers.

Any form of masking must be checked before the exercises begin. The simple question of whether the patient can still hear something in the masked ear is not sufficient. Patients can quite reliably perceive a changed hearing situation, but not whether nothing is perceived on one side.

As soon as the therapist suspects sufficient masking of the opposite ear, the patient is asked to remove the coil of the CI with which he is practicing, while the therapist continues to speak. After the coil has been reattached, the patient is asked whether they can still hear or even understand something. Only when the patient perceives absolute silence or only a possible tinnitus without the CI is the masking optimal. Otherwise, further measures must be taken and the masking checked again afterwards. The procedure should be briefly explained to the patient beforehand and accompanied by gestures during the implementation, as the patient temporarily can't hear anything during this procedure.

▶   Measures for Masking the Opposite Ear in Increasing Strength

1. If the patient wears a hearing system on the opposite side, this is first switched off and removed from the head or ear.
2. The ear gets closed with an earplug. For hearing aid wearers who have an earmold on the hearing aid, the switched-off hearing aid can be inserted and used as a substitute for an earplug.

5.1 Exercise Areas and Their Implementation

3. A capsule hearing protection is worn over the earplugs; these are available in different strengths.
4. If the spatial conditions allow, a greater distance of several meters is put between the patient and the therapist, and a microphone is used for direct streaming to the CI.

In addition, a noise could also be played in the ear. This method should be used with great caution, as it means a huge acoustic overload for the patient, and the increased demand for concentration can distort the auditory training result.

Not with every patient an optimal masking can be achieved. Especially, SSD patients often report still being able to hear parts of the language, sometimes even understand it. If the therapist's speech is only recognized but not understood, this can be accepted as optimal masking, but must be taken into account in the feedback for the adjustment of the sound processor. Alternatively, exercises can initially be used via an audio source (Sect. 3.3.2). If the patient still understands the therapist, training via a direct connection to an audio source or via video chat is recommended (Sect. 3.3.3). At the latest, with exercises in noise, understanding via the masked ear is significantly more difficult due to the additional noise level in the room. Therefore, especially with SSD patients, the masking should be checked again in this situation in order to possibly be able to switch to live-voice.

5.1.2.3 Volume Setting

If the other side is sufficiently masked, the volume setting with the CI is checked. Often, the volume is too low as soon as the information from the second side isn't available due to the masking. But even with deafness on the other side, the volume may not be sufficient. If the patient is permanently supplied with too little volume, further progress can only be made inadequately, as understanding speech is linked to a sufficient input volume. This becomes visible in the hearing test when increased volume in speech audiometry can also be understood better (Zeh and Baumann 2015) or when the assistance of speaking "Louder" in auditory training provides better results. The goal is a setting in which the therapist's speech is perceived as strong, but still pleasantly loud. This also corresponds to the target setting of the C-Level during the fitting. The patient is asked to slowly increase the volume until this target setting is reached. Meanwhile, the therapist speaks at normal volume. It is possible that the patient's adjustable maximum volume has been reached, so that it is necessary to switch to a louder program or to change the settings in a fitting as soon as possible.

▶ If it is assumed that the patient cannot understand the instructions during the volume adjustment, the procedure must be discussed before the other side is masked.

If it turns out during the exercise that the volume should be a bit higher, this can be adjusted during the course of the auditory training session. A strong and rapid volume adjustment is usually only necessary in the first few weeks. If the patient still reports needing significantly more volume after several fittings and therapies, consultation with the CI technician should be held.

At the end of each training session, the masking of the other side is reversed, which leads to a significantly higher overall volume for the patient. In this case, the previously adjusted volume can be reduced to a tolerable level. Often, patients describe the higher volume as pleasant and want to keep it.

5.1.2.4 Understanding Without Lip-Seeing

If both conversation partners can also see each other in communication, the acoustic information is always supplemented by visual one's. The worse the hearing is, the more important the visual information becomes. In addition to gestures and facial expressions, specifically, the mouth shapes of individual sounds, so-called kinemes, provide this additional visual information (Lindner 1999, p. 108). This leads to the fact that with increasing duration of hearing loss, the abilities in lip-seeing become better and better. Especially since the pandemic in 2020 and the face mask requirement, it has become clear that not only the mouth shape, but indeed the entire area between the hairline and the larynx is observed. Despite the therapist wearing a mask, it is usually easier for patients to understand if they look at the therapist during the exercise instead of looking away. To ensure that only listening and understanding, and not lip-seeing, is trained in auditory training, at least the mouth shape must be excluded (Heinemann 2014, p. 23; Diller 1997, p. 91). It is even more effective to prevent the view of the entire head and neck area of the therapist. In addition, the patient should become more independent of visual information through improved understanding.

Some therapists use frames covered with speaker fabric in therapy to hold them in front of their mouths or face when speaking. This makes lip-seeing more difficult, but, similar to a face mask, it can provide visual information in understanding. If the patient turns to the side to look away, this is also unsuitable due to possible directional characteristics in the setting of the sound processor and the visual perception in the corner of the eye. Lip-seeing is most reliably excluded when the patient is asked to lower their gaze.

LipReading vs. Lip-Seeing

"Lipreading" or "reading from the lips" are common phrases when describing that someone includes the mouth shape to a greater extent in understanding. However, the word "reading" implies that every speech sound is clearly visually recognizable, just like the letters when reading. This would mean that everything verbally spoken can be understood without audible sounds, so we only need the mouth shape. However, this does not correspond to reality. Humans are only able to see some speech sounds and then supplement the acoustic information with the visual. Therefore, it's better to speak of "lip-seeing."

5.1.2.5 Recognizing Patient Fatigue

The exercises in auditory training cost the patients a lot of energy and require a high level of concentration. If clear exhaustion and fatigue are noticed in the exercise, continuation for the sake of practice is not appropriate. Fatigue is particularly noticeable through sudden drops in performance during exercise or general physical signs of a loss of concentration.

Often, it is enough to take a short break or to revert to an easier or nonlinguistic exercise. Rarely, in the first few weeks, the cognitive demand can be so high that the patient's capacities are completely exhausted and the exercise part of the respective training session should be ended.

5.1.2.6 Interdisciplinary Exchange with CI Technicians

Only in a professional exchange can an optimal fitting of the sound processor be achieved. Any abnormalities should therefore always be communicated promptly with the audiological department staff of the CI-supplying clinic (Sect. 5.3).

5.1.3 Speech Sounds and Syllables

Most patients last dealt with speech sounds and their function in their early school days. As soon as written language is learned, the concept of letters dominates. Many are not aware that speech sounds and letters are not the same, which can lead to difficulties within training, but also in relation to the fitting of the sound processor. Therefore, patient feedback in this regard should always be questioned. If training is carried out at the speech sound level, it sometimes requires an explanation as to why the sounds are pronounced differently by the therapist than initially assumed by the patients. They usually expect the naming of the letter. Therefore, the previous introduction of the sound of the speech sound used in the exercise is often necessary.

Even though words consist of strung-together syllables and these in turn consist of a sequence of speech sounds (Eisenberg 2016, p. 37), individual speech sounds do not carry any meaning. For this reason, and also in connection with the lack of coarticulation, it is of rather limited use for language comprehension. If the aim is to practice detection and discrimination, however, speech sounds are more distinct than everyday noises and offer the opportunity to perceive linguistic sound, in preparation for more complex linguistic exercise areas. In addition, individual speech sounds can provide insight into a possible frequency-specific imbalance in the setting.

Syllables, on the other hand, come much closer to linguistic reality in everyday life, as the sequence of several speech sounds requires coarticulatory processes, and, as monosyllabic words, they represent the smallest meaning-bearing unit of spoken language. As a result, syllables can be used in exercises both at the level of identification and understanding.

5.1.4 Words, Phrases, Sentences, and Texts

The more pronounced a hearing loss, the more often people have to supplement the incomplete linguistic information. Even after the CI-supply, patients must rely on this combination ability and use it as a strategy to compensate for the difficulties in perception and processing (Hahne et al. 2012, p. 1201). A frequent combination means for the patient a high cognitive effort. To reduce this, one goal of auditory training is to reduce the frequency of combinations through improved acoustic hearing and understanding. To increase language comprehension, it is most effective to train within linguistic exercise areas. In addition, language-based exercises allow precise conclusions for the fitting of the sound processor. Therefore, exercises in the area of words, phrases, sentences, and texts have a high priority in training with a CI.

Due to the abundance of written sources in everyday life, specific therapy material does not necessarily have to be procured. Whether books, magazines, newspapers, advertising brochures, package inserts, or the list of ingredients on a pack of cookies, almost any material can be used in auditory training. Anyone who sharpens their eye for potential exercise materials in everyday life can offer their patients a very varied therapy in terms of content and at the same time creates again and again an occasion for an exchange, to work towards the goal of improved everyday communication.

5.1.5 Everyday Communication

Communication is a highly complex process that combines various cognitive performances (Sect. 5.1.1). Over the course of auditory training, more and more of these performances are combined in the exercises. A prerequisite for this is a stable setting of the sound processor. An overlap of too many new demands, while the acoustic understanding has not yet been optimized, is demotivating and very exhausting for the patient.

Every day communication plays a major role for the patient from the very beginning, as it often results in one of the greatest burdens: The restricted social participation. All interventions of auditory training and fitting should aim to improve participation (DGHNO-KHC e.V. 2020). This takes time and patience, which patients do not always have due to the pressure of suffering. The approach to the level of everyday communication should therefore be clearly named and repeatedly classified in the ongoing training process.

An approach to everyday communication always consists of a combination of two integration possibilities. On the one hand, it can be integrated into specific exercises; on the other hand, it can be embedded in the conversation between the exercises. The integration into the exercises can already start from word exercises of difficulty level 2, for example, by adding the memorization of a few items to the

5.1 Exercise Areas and Their Implementation

exercise type of speaking and repeating. Outside of the exercise, various intermediate conversations offer themselves to create short and natural communication situations. Already at the beginning of the training session, the exchange about hearing experiences of the past days can be used for a short conversation with the therapist. Similarly, exercise instructions and short evaluation conversations after the exercises are suitable for a conversation modeled on everyday communication.

▶ **Tip** To continue using therapy conversations for training acoustic understanding, it is useful to additionally mask the opposite ear even outside of the exercises.

Since the patient does not cover the opposite ear in everyday life and may and should use all available means to facilitate communication, exercises without covering are also useful in the later course of training. Similarly, additional technical accessories can be used together to test their suitability for everyday use (Sect. 3.4). For this, the fitting process for optimizing acoustic understanding should be largely completed, and any hearing systems on the other side and the CI should be coordinated with each other (Fig. 5.1).

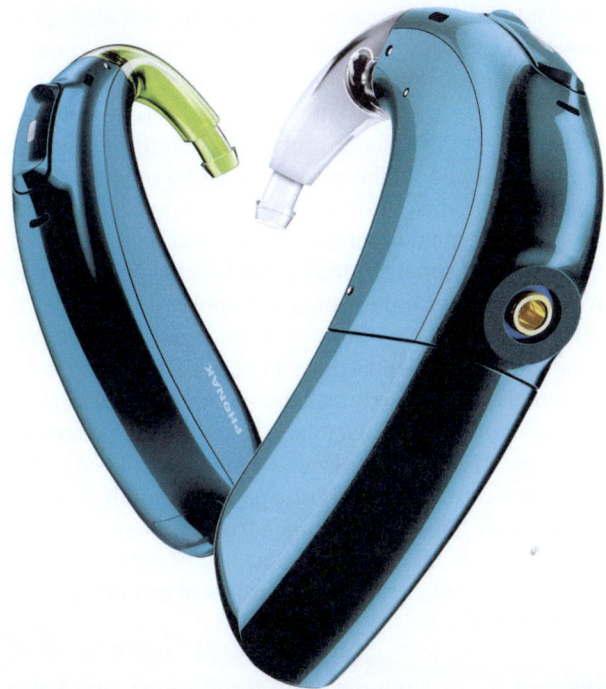

Fig. 5.1 Bimodal hearing solution consisting of hearing aid (left) and the Naída CI M (right, here without transmitter coil). (Courtesy of Advanced Bionics. All rights reserved)

Adapting Hearing Systems in Bilateral or Bimodal Supply

1. Both devices must be at their respective optimal fitting level.
2. Both devices are independently increased to the necessary volume in training. For this, the other side is temporarily masked.
3. Both devices are worn together again and equally as well as simultaneously (either increasing or decreasing both sides) in volume corrected until the sound is pleasant when hearing on both sides.

In order to orient the training as closely as possible to the patient's everyday life at this point, specific situations, such as the workplace, can be asked about. If the patient works in an environment that can be modelled for the exercise, this should be used to support the patient as specifically as possible.

5.1.6 Hearing and Understanding in Noise

The environment is strongly characterized by various noises. How these are perceived depends on the respective situation, the noise itself, and the individual condition of a person. If something is to be heard or understood in this environment, it can be disturbed by other noises. Therefore, we also speak of background noise. The so-called useful sound, such as the language in communication, can be impaired by the background noise or sometimes not be perceptible at all (Fellbaum 2012, p. 118). Nevertheless, in many situations, the normal-hearing human is able to separate background noise from useful sound as long as the noise does not completely cover the useful sound. In the case of a hearing impairment, it is difficult or impossible to do this at all. This is due to the changed perception, on the one hand, and the limited acoustic information intake, on the other.

After a CI supply, initially, the hearing and understanding in trained in an environment with as little background noise as possible. However, since this does not reflect the noise environment of everyday life, the transition to background noise should occur as soon as the patient understands speech in a quiet environment well. Experience has shown that the addition of background noises is beneficial for a large part of the patients, as soon as sentence exercises with difficulty level 4 to text exercises with difficulty level 3 can be completed with little assistance.

To avoid overwhelming the patient, a gradual increase in the complexity of the background noise is recommended. The same speech material is used as for the exercises in silence, and the sequence of exercises remains the same. As a rule, the start can be made with word exercises of difficulty level 3 to sentence exercises with difficulty level 2.

Increase in the Complexity of the Background Noise

1. Understanding with constant background noise from one direction and from one speaker without impulse noise.

5.1 Exercise Areas and Their Implementation

2. Understanding with various constant noises from multiple directions and from speakers without impulse noise (e.g., white noise, plus a rather monotonous voice such as an audiobook)
3. Understanding with various constant noises from multiple directions and from speakers with impulse noise (e.g., construction site noises, plus a dialogue (e.g., podcast) or radio play).
4. Understanding in a real situation with moderate background noise (e.g., in a foyer/an entrance hall with little public traffic, a little-visited café, a garden).
5. Understanding in a real situation with various noise sources that are different in volume and contain impulse noise (e.g., street noise, a well-visited foyer).

When first approaching background noise through a speaker, it should be asked whether the patient can hear the noise and what it sounds like to him. In addition, the volume should be set at a level where the therapist's speech is still clearly audible. The volume can then be adjusted again and again within the exercise situation. Unknown noises cause discomfort and distract; noises that can be assigned are easier to ignore. It is therefore important to let the patients describe what noises they hear. The therapist can then point out further noises and give another opportunity to listen. Impulse noise usually only arises during an exercise situation. This can then be briefly discussed and assigned to a source by the therapist.

In complex background noise situations, it is important to let the patient first explore the noise environment in its entirety. This gives the patient the opportunity to get used to the acoustic conditions. The background noise must first be recognized by the patient as such in order to be able to differentiate speech from it. It should be noted that constant, continuous noises (e.g., ventilation) are easier to ignore than impulse noises (e.g., the slamming of a door).

Practicing in background noise not only has a great benefit for the patient's everyday life, but background noise programs can also be tried out, and various programs can be comparatively tested for their suitability in background noise.

▶   Programs specifically designed for background noise always require testing in real background noise situations. If background noise and useful sound are played via a direct connection of the sound processor to an audio source, the stored directional characteristics do not apply (Sect. 1.7.2).

5.1.7 Making Phone Calls

Being able to use the telephone again or better than before is a frequent wish of people who are affected by hearing loss or deafness on both sides. Not being able to use the phone harbours existential risks, such as the possible loss of a job if you have to use the phone at work (Braun 2016).

For some, the last phone call was years ago. Accordingly, there are often associated reservations and fears. This means that honest and realistic advice regarding expectations is essential. In conventional phone calls, only acoustic perception is available; additional information, such as lip-seeing, facial expressions, and gestures, cannot be relied upon. This makes using the telephone in everyday life a challenging exercise content. Therefore, it should not be made a therapy topic too early. As soon as there are no major abnormalities of the fine-tuning in the setting of the sound processor and the patient correctly repeats sentences of higher complexity levels in exercises with little or no assistance, it can be assumed that he also understands something on the phone. The limits of what is possible in this case, however, depend not only on the patient's prerequisites but also on the technical conditions.

The first attempt at a phone call is often exciting for patients. The joint, successive approach has priority in this situation. It is recommended to initially refrain from using additional technical accessories and to start with conventional phone calls by holding the speaker of the phone to the ear.

The therapist and the patient first choose a phone. The patient's private mobile phone is usually a good choice. Since the patient no longer receives sound through the ear canal, but through the sound processor microphones, he is guided to find the position (Heinemann 2014, p. 28).

Example

Therapist: "We are going to try making a phone call together now. We start simply by holding the speaker of the phone in front of the ear. Since you are now not hearing through the normal way, but through your microphones on the sound processor, the usual phone position may need to be slightly altered. After picking up, hold the phone normally in front of the ear and then move it a few centimeters upwards. Then move the phone back and forth in front of the ear or sound processor in different directions until you find the position where you hear the clearest and strongest." ◄

At this point, the patient does not yet need to understand anything on the phone. The least pressure arises when the procedure is first tested with a signal tone or noise. The dial tone when picking up, without dialing a number, is suitable for this. If this is not possible via the mobile phone, the therapist can call the patient and, after picking up, lightly stroke her phone's microphone with her finger, so that a rustling noise can be heard by the patient. This is only possible if the patient does not find the noise unpleasant. Once the patient confirms that they have found a good listening position, the therapist asks about the volume. This should be set so that the signal or noise is strong, but not uncomfortably loud. If necessary, the volume may need to be adjusted. The therapist remains in the room during the trial.

The procedure is then repeated with speech. The therapist announces to leave the room during the next call and continue to speak. The patient's task is to find the position again where the hearing sounds most pleasant and to check the volume. If the patient signals that they can already understand something, the therapist can try to ask simple questions at this point. These questions can, e.g., be about the sound or volume. After hanging up, the situation is briefly discussed.

5.1 Exercise Areas and Their Implementation

▶ With single-unit processors, making phone calls via the sound processor microphones is impractical. Holding the phone further away from the ear feels very unusual or unnatural, and the sound processor often falls off. These patients usually prefer to make phone calls via alternative connections.

As soon as it becomes clear to the patient that they can hear and understand some things, other aspects can be added, such as testing different phones or alternative forms of connection to the phone. How long and intensively phone exercises are carried out afterwards depends on the patient's needs; often, a joint first trial is enough to give a stimulus for independent training at home. This can then be supplemented by concrete suggestions for making phone calls in everyday life.

Making Phone Calls in Everyday Life with Increasing Demands

1. Dial numbers with computer-based call acceptance
2. Test phones at home with a familiar person according to the procedure in therapy, and possibly practice with material from therapy through speaking and repeating (both phone partners are in the same living space, but different rooms).
3. Arrange short phone calls with known people whose voices are familiar.
4. Arrange longer phone calls with known people whose voices are familiar.
5. Make short phone calls outside of the circle of friends and family, e.g., to make appointments.
6. Pick up the phone while another person is present who can take over.
7. Pick up the phone while no one else is present.

In this context, the patient should deal with the question of how they want to secure communication on the phone and react to communication difficulties. Depending on the point of acceptance of the disability the patient is at, this sometimes requires courage and overcoming, as it often becomes necessary to reveal one's own hearing impairment. At this point, auditory training and audio therapy overlap.

If the patient generally has difficulties in accepting their disability, they will show up in this situation and may require audio therapeutic accompaniment. In this case, for example, inpatient rehab can be considered, and the practice area of making phone calls can be moved to rehab.

If telephoning with the CI proves to be very difficult without additional technical accessories, special telephones or the connection of additional technical accessories are used (Sect. 3.4). A further attempt at a later stage of therapy is also conceivable.

▶ **Tip** Video calls offer people with a hearing impairment the opportunity to also include the mouth shape and facial expressions of the conversation partner.

There are apps that enable live translation of phone calls. These can differ from country to country.

5.1.8 Noises

A noise is defined as a non-periodic sound event (Lehnhardt 2009, p. 3), which also includes language. The crucial difference between background noise and language is that both can be heard and assigned, but only language comes with a significantly higher requirement of content understanding.

▶ **Tip** With a CI, the perception of noise at the beginning of the fitting process sometimes leads to patients feeling that they can hear everything except language. What is often meant by this is that they hear a lot, but do not yet understand language well enough.

As soon as the sound processor is fitted and switched on for the first time, patients perceive noises. From this moment on, an acoustic rediscovery of their environment begins. The biggest challenge with the CI is to perceive background noises as such and ultimately to differentiate them from the noise of language. Even during the initial fitting, it can often be impressively observed what this means for the patients and how they pause with every movement because it causes a noise. Especially patients who have lived with a hearing loss or deafness for a long time are surprised when they hear their hands brushing over their clothes, the chair scraping across the floor, and the zipper on the jacket is almost loud. This rediscovery of the environment will also continue in everyday life and will require a lot of concentration and attention from the patient. Many describe tiring quickly during this time, which is understandable due to the high number of new acoustic stimuli.

Anyone who has ever been surprised by an unfamiliar noise in their own home knows the brief moment of discomfort it triggers. To reduce this permanent stress for the CI user, patients can initially be sent home with the task of investigating their familiar environment for noises. In order to therapeutically accompany the patient and get a first impression of the usefulness of the sound processor's settings, it should be asked at the beginning of the training session which noises the patient was able to hear in the past few days, which noises were possibly surprising or also disturbing, or unpleasant.

▶ **Tip** Some noises are perceived by patients as very dominant and intense. This is not always an indication of a problem in the setting. Many patients are not aware of how loud some noises are and how quickly speech can be obscured by background noise. Here, it can help to objectify and visualize the hearing impression. For example, apps for measuring decibels can give an idea of how close background noise intensity and speech intensity are to each other. Although these apps only allow for an approximate assessment, they are usually sufficient for orientation.

Even though noises have a high value in the patient's everyday life, this area should not take up too much space in auditory training. The depiction of everyday noises during training is not possible in the same way as in the patient's actual everyday life. The daily confrontation with noise is so ubiquitous that the presentation via audio sources, as is often used in auditory training for this purpose, does not do it justice. In addition, many noises available on CDs or in hearing programs are not relevant to everyday life or clearly assignable. Similarly, for example, Shafiro et al. (2015, p. 516) in a study found no significant advantage in generalized noise identification, outside of the noises that were trained, and a resulting profit in speech understanding. This makes exercises for noise identification rather unsuitable for achieving greater hearing success. Also, in order to effectively pursue the goal of optimal sound processor adjustment, frequency-specific verification in the exercises is required. The sound of speech is much better suited for this. Nevertheless, sounds can be used in this context as an additional way of reassuring the therapist's observation (Sect. 5.3).

This by no means implies the exclusion of the area "noises" from auditory training. Not feeling the pressure to have to understand something can, for example, create the advantage for long-deaf or hard-of-hearing people of a gentle introduction to auditory training. When using nonlinguistic noises, the measure is therefore decisive. The nonlinguistic area can have an important benefit when used purposefully, but should not become the focus, as the main emphasis is on understanding speech.

5.1.9 Tones

Music is an emotionally charged topic for many people. For people with hearing loss in general and specifically for CI patients, the altered sound of music is sometimes hard to bear. This often leads to the desire to practice listening to music. Discrimination exercises in the area of tones are a first step towards a new enjoyment of music. In this process, patients learn how different tones on different instruments sound. Although there are patients who are generally able to distinguish between two tones that are up to a semitone apart (Wang et al. 2011), different instruments can also be perceived differently. Fuller et al. (2018) found, for example, that melodic progressions on the piano were more difficult to follow than on the organ.

Just like working with individual speech sounds and noises, the discrimination of tones can provide insights into the setting of the sound processor. However, great caution is required here with regard to different results depending on the instrument. Therefore, other practice material should be preferred to tones.

5.1.10 Melody and Music

Once the patient has gained an impression of the area of tones of how different instruments sound at different pitches, listening to music can be increasingly broadened and brought closer and closer to the listening of a piece of music. Despite all efforts, music will always sound somewhat different from how it does with a normal ear. The goal is therefore not to achieve the state before the CI, but rather to acquire a new way of dealing with music. Accepting this and allowing the new sound perception requires a lot from the patient.

A connection between improved speech understanding after training in the area of melody has been suspected time and again in the past. So far, there is no satisfactory evidence for this. For example, Lo et al. (2015) were able to find parallels to improvements in the identification of consonants as well as interrogative and declarative sentences, but no changes in understanding in noise. Fuller et al. also found no interactions in 2018 between regular exercise with melodic progressions and a change in word and sentence perception.

5.1.11 Voices

In the first weeks after the initial fitting, many patients find the sound of a CI to be unnatural. Voices are often described as squeaky, like Mickey Mouse, or electronic, like a robot. At this point, it usually makes no difference who is speaking. All people sound very similar or even the same. The further the acclimatization to the CI and the fitting of the sound processor progress, the better voices can be distinguished from each other, and the more natural the sound gradually becomes. Experience has shown that it often takes several months for a normal and natural sound to develop. It is not uncommon for speech understanding to be possible at a high level before this. Since the development of the sound is very much dependent on acclimatization, the therapist, along with close people, is often one of the first people who can be identified by the patient by voice. The extent of familiarization with the therapist's voice becomes particularly clear when another therapist takes over or trainees accompany the auditory training and help to shape the exercises. It is normal for a temporary deterioration in understanding the exercises to occur in such cases, which usually only lasts a few minutes.

If one wants to practice with the patient to discriminate and identify voices, this should be postponed at least until the first weeks after the initial fitting. Otherwise, this could lead to frustration. The goal of these exercises is primarily to deal with the subtleties of sound perception and a more relaxed approach to unknown speakers. In addition, the knowledge of being able to get used to voices can give patients self-confidence and security for communication with strangers. Thus, for patients in this exercise area, there is a relevant everyday context.

5.1.12 Spatial Hearing

As soon as an adult person starts to become hard of hearing, they notice increasing difficulties in localizing noises or voices. Patients report with high reliability turning in the wrong direction or around their own axis as soon as they hear something in the distance. This means a loss of control, which in some situations, such as in traffic, can even be life-threatening. To reliably determine a direction based on acoustic information, two healthy ears are needed. In the case of hearing loss, this ability decreases the more pronounced the hearing loss is and the more different both ears are in their function (Heinemann 2014, p. 29). In a study, in which SSD patients heard speech next to and in front of them from seven different directions, the CI-supplied patients performed best compared to patients with other monaural supply options (e.g., a CROS system) and could also improve their spatial hearing compared to monaural hearing with the healthy ear (Arndt et al. 2011). The sentences were presented in a quiet environment, and a selection of possible directions was given. In such experimental setups, results are well captured for very specific situations, but do not allow reliable conclusions about the diverse situations of the patient's everyday life. The situations in which patients often find themselves are characterized by many noises coming from various directions and distances, and varying greatly in their duration and volume. This makes localization, regardless of the treatment of hearing loss, so difficult and also hard to train. Therefore, expectations in this area should be kept low.

It is conceivable to limit therapy to the four directions: front, back, left, and right. In addition, the therapist must consider that impulse noise is hardly locatable due to its short duration, so longer-lasting or repeating noises are more suitable for practice. If the patient perceives particularly well from one direction, he can help by turning his head back and forth to confirm the direction. Furthermore, exercises for spatial hearing should only be carried out with the best possible bilateral supply, i.e., without masking. For quiet exercises in which the therapist makes the sounds themselves (e.g., clapping, snapping), it must also be ensured that the patient cannot hear the direction in which the therapist is moving when changing position.

Exercise Options in the Area of Spatial Hearing

1. Joint comparison of how a noise sounds from different directions, where the patient knows the direction. For this, the patient can change his position to the noise source, or the therapist can present the noise from different directions.
2. Guide the patient to practice perceiving noises from his domestic environment from different directions (see 1.).
3. Exercise in quiet from four directions with noises or speech, while the patient closes their eyes. The patient names or indicates the direction in which they suspect the sound is coming from.
4. Exercise in moderate background noise from four directions with noises or speech, while the patient closes their eyes. The patient names or indicates the direction in which they suspect the sound is coming from.

5. Exploring a noisy situation with eyes closed, indicating which sounds can be heard from where, e.g., before starting a speech-based exercise with background noise.

5.1.13 Independent Training at Home

To achieve sufficient acclimatization to the CI and thereby improve understanding, the patient must independently continue the training in their everyday life. This is, according to a survey by Anton and Otero (2018, p. 57), also the consensus of therapists in practice. While independent training at home serves general familiarization and repetition, auditory training works on specific problems.

First, and this is a prerequisite for hearing success, the patient must wear the CI regularly. The recommended wearing time is at least 8 hours a day. To increase the acclimatization effect over time, the patient can be advised to mask the opposite side as often and as well as possible in everyday life.

▶ In the everyday life of many patients, masking the opposite side is difficult to implement and should not be expected per se. It is important to communicate clearly that it must be appropriate to the situation and the condition of the patient and must not lead to overexertion. The urgency of regular wearing of the CI, however, must be clearly expressed and demanded.

Furthermore, there is the possibility of performing specific exercises. A distinction is made between exercises that the patient performs alone and exercises that relatives or friends perform with them.

If the patient practices alone, this creates the advantage of person-independent and partially location-independent training. On the other hand, only a limited amount of material and no live-voice speaker is available. The frequency is determined by the capacities of the patient.

Possibilities of Independent Training at Home
1. Listening to and/or reading along with audiobooks
2. Exercise offers from CI manufacturers online
3. Listening to podcasts
4. Online available and current news in picture and/or sound
5. Apps for CI users in the respective national language

When practicing together with relatives or friends, any speech material can be converted into exercise material. These can be materials from auditory training, newspapers and magazines, books, etc. To avoid overwhelming the patient and relatives, specific exercises should be discussed.

▶ Relatives and friends are not therapists. Joint exercises are only for acclimatization or repetition and should not be felt as a duty by either side. It may be necessary to repeatedly discuss this with patients and relatives.

5.2 Feedback to the Patient

Patients with hearing loss often feel insecure in communication, which is why the therapy with CI aims to reduce doubts and insecurities in communication for the patients. The uncertainty in dealing with one's own abilities and limits, especially in terms of communication, arises mainly from not knowing what was misunderstood or perhaps not heard at all, and the experiences the patient has had in communication with others as a result. The therapist should create a place and an atmosphere that gives the patient a sense of security and the feeling of being able to communicate on an equal footing despite the hearing impairment. To achieve this, the therapist must not fall into a childish way of speaking or a clear over-articulation. Hearing loss causes problems in acoustic understanding, not in thinking.

This means that the therapist gives the patient appreciative feedback that they may rarely hear in everyday life. This can also be the confrontation with an obvious misunderstanding after the patient has answered past the question. But the therapist also encourages asking regularly and to secure communication by having an open and honest exchange about the fact that the therapist neither judges nor evaluates. In auditory training, there is always room for the patient to experiment with his communication behavior. This claim must be met throughout the entire training, both during the exercise situation and the initial conversation or in evaluation discussions at the end of an exercise.

Within the exercises, a purely acoustic understanding is enforced, without the patient primarily involving the mouth shape (Sect. 5.1.2). In case of errors, feedback is given within the framework of various assistances, which are described in detail in Sect. 5.2.1. In addition, feedback on the correctness should ideally be given after each answer by the patient, regardless of whether the answer was correct or not. The feedback can range from a visual, nonverbal hint like a thumbs up or a negating moving index finger in the patient's field of vision, to differentiated verbal reactions, such as "Yes, very good, now you have been able to understand the [m] at the beginning of the word correctly." or "That was almost correct, only the word at the end sounds a bit different." (Montano and Spitzer 2021, p. 518). This can result in overlaps with some assistance. Just like the assistance, other feedback in the exercise can be introduced successively. This way, the patient can gradually get used to different variants and is once again encouraged that communication in the training setting is always secured. Exceptions are patients who have already reached a high level and need very little to no assistance. They are sometimes already so confident that not every answer needs to be confirmed. However, assistance in case of not understanding correctly should still be applied.

At the end of a training session, a brief evaluation is made together with the patient of what worked well and in which areas further exercises or possibly a fitting of the sound processor are necessary. To better understand where problems still exist, feedback is given from both sides. At the beginning, the patient may still find it difficult to come to a differentiated statement and will express themselves rather unspecifically. To give the patient a clearer picture of the current status, this assessment is supplemented therapeutically. The patient's assessment is also an instrument for the therapist to find out how realistically improvements and limits of the supply are seen (Sect. 2.3.1).

5.2.1 Assisting Techniques During the Exercise

Each exercise can be spontaneously simplified using various assisting techniques. The choice of assistance is based on the individual's needed support and the structure of the exercise. Not every assisting technique is suitable for every patient or for every exercise. Additionally, the needs of the patient must always be taken into account.

The following are listed, described, and classified according to their degree of strength. The scale is set from 1 to 3, where "1" indicates a low, "2" a medium, and "3" a high degree of strength and thus also support. If one cannot do without medium or strong support in an exercise, the difficulty level of the exercise is not initially changed or possibly even reduced in order not to overwhelm the patient. In practice, combinations of different assisting techniques are often used, which is not a problem in the course of the exercise. In addition, after a few exercises and with increasing experience, it quickly becomes apparent which assisting techniques or combinations of them are actually supportive for the individual patient.

5.2.1.1 Assisting Technique Level 1
Repetition Without Changing the Pronunciation of the Item
After the first demonstration, repeating in the same way is a very simple assisting technique and can be used in any exercise. Depending on the patient's frustration tolerance, the target item is repeated several times. The sense of achievement of understanding something after repetition is greater for the patient than after an assisting technique.

Louder
A louder pronunciation should be used with caution and is not equivalent to extremely loud speaking or shouting, but rather to raising the voice slightly. The attempt at very loud pronunciation leads to distortions in the speech sound and is therefore not helpful for the patient. However, a slightly louder presentation of the target item can lead to better understanding if the basic volume setting of the sound processor is too low. This assistance is suitable for all exercises. The patient may have difficulty assessing the perceived volume, so even adjusting the volume at the beginning of the training session may not have been sufficient. If better

communication is observed when the voice is raised, the patient should be made aware of this, and the volume on the sound processor should be increased under guidance.

Orientation to the Patient's Dialect
It is easier with the CI to understand things to which one was already accustomed in terms of sound and content before the hearing loss. Since the training should always be carried out in standard language (without the influence of accents or dialects), this can lead to difficulties with individual words for patients who speak a dialect. For the therapist, this by no means implies the need to acquire the dialect. It is about orienting oneself to what the patient brings with them. This primarily refers to features of prosody. If variations in language are noticed in auditory training, the therapist can adopt these as an assistance, especially for words and short sentences.

> **Example**
>
> *Therapist*: "She became [ˈθɜːd]." ("th" in Standard English)
> *Patient*: "She became a sherd?!"
> *Therapist*: "No, she became [tɜːd]." ("t" instead of "th", e.g., with an Irish accent) ◀

Position in the Word or Position in the Phrase/Sentence
Patients who have already achieved good speech understanding with their CI can better focus on the position of the erroneous speech sound or the corresponding letter, or the erroneous word, when listening again with a hint to the position. It often happens that the subsequent repetition is combined with other assisting techniques, such as emphasis or slightly slower speaking of the corresponding speech sound or word.

> **Example**
>
> *Specific naming of the sound position*: "The first speech sound is different."
> *Broader word position*: "The word in the middle is not quite right yet." ◀

5.2.1.2 Assisting Technique Level 2
Syllabic
Syllabic speaking is particularly suitable for words and makes it easier for the patient to perceive a word in its entirety. The use of this assistance is particularly useful when syllables are often omitted while repeating. Very short pauses are made after each syllable, but they should not be too long and unnatural in order not to alienate the word too much. It is only about emphasizing the word structure and rhythm.

Slower
Speaking slower leads to a reduction in speaking pace and often to a clearer articulation. This gives the patient time to understand and process. Especially with

sentences or texts, it can happen that the patient does not understand a word at the beginning of the utterance and lingers there mentally. Everything said afterwards is often not well captured. The sound of individual words should be maintained. Originally, short-spoken speech sounds are not stretched, and likewise, the prosody of an utterance is not changed.

Change of the Word Form
If a patient does not understand a word after repeated repetition, it may be due to the sound composition or the length of the word. Perhaps a wrong word was understood, which is now heard over and over again. In such a case, it helps to change the word. This can be done by extending the word or by changing the sound. Possible is an extension to a compound noun, declination, conjugation, or the variation of the tense of a word.

> **Example**
>
> *Original word*: rain
> *Extension possibilities*: rainforest; raining ◀

Expand to Phrase/Sentence
Similar to changing the word form, it can be helpful to increase the number of words or to give an item a contextual connection.

If a patient can already understand simple sentences, a word can be embedded in a phrase or a sentence, or a phrase in a sentence. For this, idioms and phrases are suitable. If there is no suitable idiom or phrase, a newly formed phrase or a newly formed sentence is used. This also increases the difficulty level or reduces the strength of the assistance. A new sentence should not be too long, as the target item might get lost among the additional information.

> **Example**
>
> *Original word*: gold
> *Extension possibilities:*
> Silver and gold.
> A necklace made of gold.
> Gold is very valuable.
> As good as gold. ◀

Comparison
If a patient repeatedly understands the same wrong utterance, it becomes difficult for them to understand anything else, as what they have supposedly understood cannot simply be reversed. You can then announce to the patient to first say the wrongly understood word and then the target item to allow a comparison. Often, this leads to something other than the wrong utterance being perceived. This assisting technique is only suitable for items of limited length, i.e., a maximum of one short sentence. Both utterances together can otherwise exceed the memory span.

5.2 Feedback to the Patient

> **Example**
>
> *Starting word*: sheep
> *Formulation possibilities*:
> "I will say the word that you have understood and then the correct word. sleep [short pause] sheep."
> "I say both words one after the other, first the wrong one and then the right one. sleep [short pause] sheep." ◄

▶ **Tip** Asking whether both words sound exactly the same or whether the patient was able to perceive a difference can provide information about discrepancies in the setting of the sound processor or about getting used to the sound. If the same speech sounds are often involved, these should be noted for the fitting of the sound processor.

Initial Speech Sound
Especially when the initial speech sound that has been understood is very far away from the actual speech sound of the target word, it makes sense to say the misunderstood speech sound. This is spoken as a speech sound and not as a letter.

> **Example**
>
> *Therapist*: "The word begins with [f]." or "At the beginning you hear a [p]." ◄

Initial Letter
Some patients find it difficult to understand the difference between letters and speech sounds, so the initial letter is used instead of the speech sound. The procedure is the same as for the initial speech sound, but with letters, there is the additional possibility of writing it down or using letter cards. A simple extension to sentences is also possible. For this, the initial letters of all words in the sentence are laid out as cards or written down. With letter cards, this assisting technique can be gradually withdrawn by continuing to lay out all letter cards, but some are presented covered up. As soon as the patient says the correct word, the letter is uncovered.

For patients competent in sign language, the letter can be spelled according to the finger alphabet. If you do not know the finger alphabet yourself, a picture of the finger position can be shown.

▶ **Tip** Suitable materials could be magnetic letter tiles or letter tiles from the game "Scrabble."

Rhythmic Tapping
Similar to syllabic speaking, this assisting technique can represent a number nonverbally. For this, the rhythm is quietly tapped on the table in the patient's field of vision with the finger. In this way, syllables of a word, words of a phrase, or words

of a sentence can be represented. Since this is a nonverbal assistance, it is particularly suitable for CI users with still low language comprehension.

Pointing to Spoken Words
A very simple exercise can be reading along with sentences or short texts. If patients are unable to follow sentences or texts despite visual representation, the therapist initially follows the spoken words with their finger. Similarly, the assisting technique of the initial letters can be extended to the sentence level. The initial letters of all words in the sentence are laid out in the correct order on the table. Then, the letter is pointed to, to which the corresponding word is currently being said.

Stretching Speech Sounds
Stretching sounds is an assistance that is particularly suitable for exercises with speech sounds, syllables, and words. In this case, the sound that was not correctly understood is held for a short time. This assistance is suitable for any speech sound position and all speech sounds that can be stretched.

Emphasizing Speech Sounds in a Word or Words in a Phrase/Sentence
If a speech sound within a word is not correctly repeated, the word can be mentioned again, and the incorrectly repeated speech sound emphasized. This applies to speech sounds that cannot be stretched and is valid for exercises with words, phrases, or sentences. In a phrase/sentence, not the entire target item, but only the affected word is repeated, and the incorrect speech sound is emphasized, so one temporarily moves from the phrase or sentence level to the word level.

If a word within a phrase/sentence is not only changed in one speech sound, but completely different, the phrase or sentence is repeated completely, and the misunderstood word is emphasized.

With this assisting technique, there are often overlaps with speaking louder.

Explicit Pronunciation
In phonetics, different variants of pronunciation are distinguished. The most common form in everyday communication is the colloquial pronunciation, which is the desired pronunciation variant in auditory training. It is closest to reality and is therefore particularly relevant for the CI user. However, this type of pronunciation is also particularly challenging for people with hearing loss. Explicit pronunciation can be used as a help to slowly approach the colloquial pronunciation.

Explicit pronunciation is characterized by various properties:

1. The words are pronounced individually and thus independently of previous or subsequent pronunciation
2. Each sound of a word is spoken with all its functional and articulatory features
3. All syllables are taken into account in pronunciation, so that each syllable has an audible vowel as the syllable nucleus
4. The pronunciation is in normal emphasis (cf. Eisenberg 2016, 51 ff.)

5.2 Feedback to the Patient

The demarcation from over-articulation, as it occurs, for example, in the context of overpronunciation, is very important here, as this form of pronunciation would change what was said too much (Heinemann 2014, p. 24f.).

> **Example**
>
> *Therapist*: "[tʃIkŋ]"
> *Patient*: "[...]"
> *Therapist*: "[tʃIkən]" ◄

5.2.1.3 Assisting Technique Level 3
Giving a Choice
If an exercise is only auditory, it can be converted into a visual exercise by providing a selection of written or picture cards. The scope of the selection should range between three and eight items. This way, a randomly correct selection can be better excluded and the patient can still overview all the options. This assistance can be well implemented at the word and phrase level or in exercises with short sentences.

Reducing Selection
To make a visual exercise easier, the already given selection of items can be reduced. The total amount should not be less than three to better exclude a randomly correct selection. The closer the general sound and the more similar the length of all remaining items, the higher the remaining exercise difficulty.

Pauses in the Phrase/Sentence
When we speak, it is in a continuous flow of speech, which is interspersed with barely perceptible pauses. Longer pauses only occur when a punctuation mark, like a full stop, requires it.

Especially when relearning acoustic understanding, this leads to words merging too much, and content understanding is often no longer possible as soon as the previous word could not be understood. If utterances are complex in their length or if the patient is at the beginning of a higher difficulty level in the exercises, short pauses help to better recognize word boundaries and to better grasp the meaning. The pause should only be as long as the end of a word is recognizable, but the patient does not assume that the utterance is already complete.

Mouth Shape
In a training that is about acoustic understanding with the CI, the mouth shape should always be the last option for assistance (Sect. 4.2.3). Especially when the topic is known, a lot of information can be gleaned from the mouth shape for a large part of the patients. The correct answer is then mainly seen and no longer heard.

▶ The listed assisting techniques are especially suitable for linguistic exercise areas. For the areas of "noises," "voices," "discrimination of tones," and "melody and music," the selection is significantly limited.

Repetitions and a louder presentation are always possible. Depending on the exercise structure, a selection of items can be given or an existing selection reduced, as well as initial letters given if an explicit name or title is sought.

None of the assisting techniques used should lead to a strong alienation or change of the target item; otherwise, it cannot be excluded that the distortion of the target item led to misunderstanding. Nevertheless, items should be repeated in colloquial language after assisting as soon as the patient has understood correctly. This allows him to compare with the sound in everyday communication and creates an additional repetition.

> **Example**
>
> *Connection with positive confirmation*: "Yes, very good, the word was bouquet."
> *Present the word alone*: "Correct. I say the word [possibly repetition gesture with the index finger] again: [short pause] bouquet." ◄

Various assisting techniques should, especially for CI users who still have a severely limited understanding of speech, be introduced slowly and successively. This usually requires no explanation for the patient. Even after a short time, the difference between what is said in the context of the assistance and the new item is clearly recognizable for most, especially if praise is given after successful repetition of the target item and a short break is taken.

5.2.2 Transcript of an Exercise

To get a better picture of the use of assisting techniques, here are excerpts of an exercise sequence in the form of a transcript. The training session took place online via video chat. The patient has had the CI for several months and was last in inpatient rehab. She reports that the co-stimulation of the facial nerve (which was already known from the CI-supplying clinic) limited the possibilities of fitting the CI in rehab. The assisting techniques are in brackets behind the respective statement.

5.2.2.1 Exercise: Difficult Nonsense Sentences (Without Background Noise)

Therapist: "During the celebrations, the salami sits in the rocking chair."
Patient: "During the celebrations, the salami sits in the rocking chair."
Therapist: "Yes. Very good. [short pause] Next to the bus stop, the sour pickle waits for autumn."
Patient: [hesitant] "Oh, next to the bus stop sits the sour pickle and waits for autumn?"
Therapist: "Hmm, now I think you've added something to it, but that's not a bad thing, so..."

5.2 Feedback to the Patient

Patient: "I'm afraid that was a concentration problem."
Therapist: "Exactly. Everything I said was in there, but it's not sitting there; it's just waiting for autumn. (Comparing "sits" and "waits," the patient looks at the therapist while she says this.)
Patient: "Ah, okay" [laughs]
Therapist: "Okay, the next sentence: Under the ground lives the family of the clock."
Patient: [thinks] "Uhh...Under the ground lives the family [short pause], not sure which family."
Therapist: "Hmm, I'll say it again. Under the ground lives the family of the clock." (repetition)
Patient: "Hmm, no."
Therapist: "Under the ground lives the family of the clock." (emphasis: "of the clock")
Patient: [questioning] "of the clock?"
Therapist: [nodding] "Mhm! Under the ground lives the family of the clock."
Patient: "Under the ground lives the family of the clock."
Therapist: "Correct. Yes. [short pause] In the classroom, the mushrooms are dancing around."
Patient: "In the classroom, the mushrooms are dancing around."
Therapist: "Correct. [short pause] On the alp, the comb rides on the whisk."
Patient: [short pause] "Can I hear that one again?"
Therapist: "Yes. [short pause] On the alp, the comb rides on the whisk."
Patient: "On the alp, the, not understood, rides on the whisk."
Therapist: "On the alp, the comb rides on the whisk." (emphasis: "the comb")
Patient: "The comb?"
Therapist: "Mhm! Yes. On the alp, the comb rides on the whisk. Exactly."
Patient: "On the alp, the comb rides on the whisk."
Therapist: "Correct. [short pause] The pea soup complains about the missing frog."
Patient: [thinks] "The pea soup complains about the [short pause] missing fog?"
Therapist: "Almost correct, I'll say it again. The end sounds very similar. The pea soup complains about the missing frog." (hint at a mistake at the beginning of the item; emphasis: "frog")
Patient: "Frog!"
Therapist: "Mhm."
Patient: "Not fog, but frog."
Therapist: "Exactly, about the missing frog." (emphasis: "frog")
Patient: "Mhm."
Therapist: "In the giraffe, the moss is buried."
Patient: "Uh, that was quick!"
Therapist: "In the giraffe, the moss is buried." (repetition)
Patient: "..."
Therapist: "In the giraffe/the moss/is buried." (pauses in the sentence at "/")
Patient: "I didn't understand the beginning, the moss is buried."
Therapist: "Exactly, the second part is correct. I'll repeat the first one. In the giraffe..." (repetition of a part of the sentence)

Patient: "In the giraffe?"
Therapist: "In the giraffe, mhm!"
Patient: "In the giraffe, the moss is buried."
Therapist: "Mhm, yes! In the giraffe, the moss is buried. Correct."
[A short conversation follows about the speaking speed, which the patient perceives as very high. The therapist assures her that it is the normal speed of colloquial language and possibly a bit faster than in the previous exercises, when understanding was overall more difficult.]
Therapist: "For relaxation, the hedgehog flutes on the Emmental cheese."
Patient: "..."
Therapist: "For relaxation, the hedgehog flutes on the Emmental cheese." (repetition)
Patient: "For relaxation..."
Therapist: "Yes!"
Patient: "Something with 'fu,' the hedgehog on the Emmental cheese."
Therapist: "Exactly, very good. For relaxation, the hedgehog flutes on the Emmental cheese." (emphasis on "flutes")
Patient: "Flutes" (elongation "u")
Therapist: "Flutes" (elongation "u")
Patient: "Flutes!" (elongation "u")
Therapist: "Exactly, for relaxation, the hedgehog flutes on the Emmental cheese." (emphasis on "flutes")
Patient: "Mhm."
Therapist: "During rush hour, the cake ends its royal visit."
Patient: "During rush hour, the cake ends its, oh, I think, royal visit."
Therapist: "Exactly, correct, it's a royal visit."
Patient: [is pleased]
Therapist: "The display case clings panically to the heating blanket."
Patient: "The display case clings panically to the heating blanket."
Therapist: "Correct. [short pause] Around midnight, the newt curves through the stone bathtub."
Patient: "Around midnight, hmm..."
Therapist: "Mhm."
Patient: "Around midnight, the newt crawls through the, hmm, was it the stone bathtub?"
Therapist: "It was, but it doesn't crawl; instead, [short pause] it curves." (comparison "crawls" and "curves")
Patient: "Curves!"
Therapist: "Mhm! Around midnight, the newt curves through the stone bathtub. Exactly. [short pause] On the manhole cover, the ladle makes its bed."
Patient: "On the manhole cover, the ladle makes its bed?"
Therapist: "Mhm, yes! [short pause] The cookie rolls at high speed over the meadow."
Patient: "The cookie rolls at high speed over the meadow."
Therapist: "Yes, very good."

5.3 Feedback to the Audiology Department

In the current guideline (DGHNO-KHC e.V. 2020), the sound processor fittings and auditory training are described as the basis for the success of treatment. Lenarz (1998, p. 124) mentions the necessity of guidance for new hearing, in order to find an optimal setting of the sound processor as a result. This means there is a need for accompaniment on the path to better hearing and understanding, which can only be achieved through the collaboration between audiology and auditory training. Dillers' (2009) assumption that a "fitting team" is needed for the care of children with CI can also be transferred to adults, which Illg (2017) describes as "collaboration of all disciplines." The closer this contact is, the faster the feedback from the therapists can be implemented in the fitting (Hermann-Röttgen 2010, p. 70 f.). To get a comprehensive picture of the patient's hearing impression, the patient should always be part of this team, whose feedback is included in addition to the professional exchange. The interlocking of the disciplines is therefore a consensus, but specific indications of the content of the exchange are not mentioned.

The possibilities of technical adjustments were discussed in Sect. 1.7. However, which feedback leads to which consequence depends on the individual approach of the CI technician. The more specific the information from the patient and the therapist, the easier it is to draw conclusions for adequate audiological treatment, and the faster the patient can achieve satisfactory speech understanding.

▶ Not every required change in the sound processor setting will be tolerated by the patient. Although the improvement of speech understanding is important, the setting should always be perceived as pleasant or tolerable by the patient. If both are not compatible or the patient cannot get used to the setting, the change is made in smaller steps and in favor of acceptance at the patient's pace.

In Sect. 3.3.1, reference is made to the form "Feedback from Auditory Training for the Fitting of the Sound Processor." This can be used for documentation and is available as online material.

5.3.1 Feedback from Patients

With each fitting of the sound processor, the patient is asked about his experiences with the CI and also about abnormalities. Often, patients use this conversation to address technical difficulties or to describe general sound and noise perceptions. Some also report specific situations in which understanding was difficult. Based on this information, initial general technical adjustments can be made. In case of serious problems, however, patients should not wait for the next scheduled appointment, but should contact the implanting clinic or the supervising rehabilitation center directly. This could be, for example, failures of the sound processor or the additional technical accessories, unbearable everyday noises, or even pain in the implant area.

▶ It is important to encourage patients in auditory training to establish contact with the audiology department staff in case of uncertainties. More serious consequences are rare, but not excluded. The rule is: It is better to reinsure once too often than to take a risk. In case of doubt, only the professional staff will be able to make a well-founded assessment of the urgency of treatment.

Especially when it comes to feedback on volume setting and speech-specific abnormalities, and thus the basis for frequency-dependent fine-tuning, the assessment becomes significantly more difficult for patients. At this point, the professional expertise of the therapists is needed, who can objectify the subjective impressions of the patients and make explicit statements about understanding in the individual frequency ranges.

Example

A patient reported in therapy about his self-training. He came to the conclusion that he had difficulties understanding the letter <g>. He was asked in which context he had noticed this. As an example, he mentioned the word <gymnastics>.

Not only does this example make it clear that patients usually do not separate written and spoken language, but it also highlights the problem that arises for the adjustment from this. Although this is about the letter <g>, it is not clear which speech sound is meant. The letter <g> can be realized in different ways, e.g., as [dʒ] in <gymnastics> or as [g] in <ground>. Both sounds are assigned to different frequency ranges. In the worst case, this feedback could have led to adjusting the wrong frequency range in the fitting of the sound processor. ◀

5.3.2 Feedback from Therapists

At the beginning of a training session, the therapist also first asks about general abnormalities and peculiarities in hearing and understanding during the last few days, which they can possibly take into account in the auditory training. This can result in relevant information for the CI fitting that requires feedback. Both the patient's statement and the conclusions drawn from it during the exercises should be reported back.

Example

The patient reports that he can have much better conversations with his wife at breakfast again, but the clattering of the crockery in the morning regularly makes him flinch. The noise sometimes feels like a stab to the brain.

5.3 Feedback to the Audiology Department

The clattering of crockery creates a clinking noise. This may be loud and present in perception, but it should not hurt or cause an unpleasant feeling in the head or ear. Such observations always require feedback to the audiologist. The clattering of dishes is a high-frequency noise. In auditory training, special attention can also be paid to high-frequency sounds in speech to check the patient's feedback. For example, if the high-frequency range is too intense, the sound [s] may also be perceived as unpleasantly hissing and dominant, or the sound [f] as sharp. This can lead to confusion of speech sounds. ◄

After a short introductory conversation, the exercise part of the training begins. At the latest now, the other ear is masked and the volume is checked (Sect. 5.1.2). Each language-specific observation takes place over a course of exercises. Individual errors can and may occur. As soon as they repeat, the cause is questioned. Tables 5.1 and 5.2 provide an overview of frequently occurring problems in auditory training. Due to the individuality of each hearing care, not all possible scenarios can be considered.

In addition to frequency-dependent feedback, requests for special programs, such as louder exercise programs or noise programs, can be made from auditory training. The therapist can also communicate how well certain programs work for the patient or which programs lead to better speech understanding compared to others.

Check Observations and Conclusions from Exercises

To verify your own observations within an exercise with the patient, the assisting technique of "Comparison" can be used. If the patient hears the same item in both variants or if parts of the item are still missing, this should be addressed in the fitting

Table 5.1 The patient did not hear anything

Problem	Possible cause	Intervention
The patient hears nothing at all	Batteries are empty Sound processor is turned off The sound processor is significantly too quiet	Change batteries Turn on the sound processor Check volume Feedback on possible sound processor defect
Missing syllables (usually at the end of the word) or replacement with a shorter item	Low basic volume	Assisting technique "Louder" Check volume Feedback on too low basic volume
Missing several different speech sounds	Low basic volume	Assisting technique "Louder" Check volume Feedback on too low basic volume
Missing the same speech sound or sounds	Low frequency-specific volume Dominance of another frequency range	Feedback on unheard speech sounds or the corresponding frequency range

Table 5.2 The patient repeats something different than what was said

Problem	Possible cause	Intervention
The same speech sounds are always confused with each other	Low-frequency-specific volume Dominance of another frequency range	Feedback on confused speech sounds or the corresponding frequency range
Different speech sounds are always confused with each other	Not yet sufficient acclimatization to the fitting	Further exercises for better acclimatization
Words are replaced by completely different ones	Low attention span (the patient hears the spoken word and combines something logical for them) Not yet sufficient acclimatization to the fitting	Reduce item length Further exercises for better acclimatization

of the sound processor. If the patient can hear a difference, insufficient acclimatization to the setting is initially conceivable.

Furthermore, an exercise-independent query of the overall sound to confirm a suspicion of unbalanced frequency ranges is conceivable. This is done in conversation and without covering the mouth shape, so that the patient can better concentrate on perception than on understanding the content. With a balanced setting, speech is usually described as strong, pleasant, round, voluminous, close, and with clearly audible, but not disturbing sibilants. Ask specifically for abnormalities and give the patient a choice of descriptions.

> **Example**
>
> *"Listen more closely to the general sound while I'm talking to you. Does what I say overall sound rather dull/humming/bass-heavy, or is it hissing a lot and sounding rather thin/squeaky/not voluminous?"*
>
> If the high frequencies are underrepresented, this leads to dull or humming perceptions. If the highs are dominant, the sound will be strongly characterized by sibilants. ◄

An additional check can also be done with the help of noises that can be assigned to a frequency range. For the approximate classification, apps for frequency measurement can help. However, the patient should not be expected to identify the noise, but only the question of the noise volume should be asked. This requires well-prepared materials.

▶ **Tip** For a reliable assessment, the patient should compare the noises. For this, the noises of a noise memory game can be sorted by the patient according to the volume they perceive.

Possible Feedback to Audiology

- Patient perception in everyday life
- Irregularities in the hardware
- Basic volume
- Overall sound of speech
- Missing syllables
- Missing and confusion of speech sounds with details of specific sounds in phonetic script, or with an example word
- Dominant or underrepresented frequency ranges
- Benefits of individual programs
- Program requests for therapy

Literature

Anton y Otero, C. (2018): Patienten Outcome bei ambulanter Therapie nach Cochlea-Implantation im Hinblick auf audiologische Ergebnisse und Angaben über den Inhalt der logopädischen Therapie. Dissertation an der Universitätsklinik für Hals-Nasen-Ohrenheilkunde, Kopf- und Halschirurgie der medizinischen Fakultät der Universität Ulm

Arndt, S.; Laszig, R.; Aschendorff, A.; Beck, R.; Schild, C.; Hassepass, F. et al. (2011): Einseitige Taubheit und Cochlear-Implant-Versorgung. Audiologische Diagnostik und Ergebnisse. In: *HNO* 59 (5), S. 437–446. https://doi.org/10.1007/s00106-011-2318-8

Beyer, R.; Gerlach, R. (2011): Sprache und Denken. 1. Aufl. Wiesbaden: VS Verlag für Sozialwissenschaften (Lehrbuch)

Braun, A. (2016): Cochlea-Implantat (CI)-Rehabilitation bei postlingual ertaubten CI-Trägern. In: *Hörakustik* (9), S. 50–52

DGHNO-KHC e.V. (2020): S2K-Leitlinie. Cochlea-Implantat Versorgung: AWMF-Register (017/071)

Diller, G. (1997): Hören mit einem Cochlear-Implant. Eine Einführung. 2., veränd. Aufl. Heidelberg: Winter Programm Ed. Schindele

Diller, G. (2009): (Re)habilitation nach Versorgung mit einem Kochleaimplantat. In: *HNO* 57 (7), S. 649–656. https://doi.org/10.1007/s00106-009-1922-3

Eisenberg, Peter (2016): Duden - die Grammatik. Unentbehrlich für richtiges Deutsch. 9., vollständig überarbeitete und aktualisierte Auflage. Hg. v. Angelika Wöllstein. Berlin: Dudenverlag (Der Duden, Band 4)

Erber, Norman P. (1982): Auditory Training: Alex Graham Bell Assn for Deaf.

Fellbaum, K. (2012): Sprachverarbeitung und Sprachübertragung. 2. Aufl. Berlin, Heidelberg: Springer Vieweg

Fuller, Christina D.; Galvin, John J.; Maat, Bert; Başkent, Deniz; Free, Rolien H. (2018): Comparison of Two Music Training Approaches on Music and Speech Perception in Cochlear Implant Users. In: *Trends in hearing* 22, 2331216518765379. https://doi.org/10.1177/2331216518765379.

Hahne, A.; Wolf, A.; Müller, J.; Mürbe, D.; Friederici, A. D. (2012): Sentence comprehension in proficient adult cochlear implant users: On the vulnerability of syntax. In: *Language and Cognitive Processes* 27 (7–8), S. 1192–1204. https://doi.org/10.1080/01690965.2011.653251.

Heinemann, S. (2014): Der Weg zum neuen Hören. Aspekte der Beratung und Therapie von erwachsenen Cochlea-Implantat-Trägern. In: *Spektrum Patholinguistik* (7), S. 13–39

Hermann-Röttgen, M. (Hg.) (2010): Cochlea-Implantat. Ein Ratgeber für Betroffene und Therapeuten. 1., Aufl. Stuttgart: TRIAS

Illg, A. (2017): Rehabilitation bei Kindern und Erwachsenen. Ein Überblick. In: *HNO* 65 (7), S. 552–560. https://doi.org/10.1007/s00106-016-0311-y

Lehnhardt, E. (Hg.) (2009): Praxis der Audiometrie. 9., vollst. überarb. Aufl. Stuttgart: Thieme

Lenarz, T. (Hg.) (1998): Cochlea-Implantat. Ein praktischer Leitfaden für die Versorgung von Kindern und Erwachsenen. Berlin: Springer.

Lindner, G. (1999): Absehen - der andere Weg zum Sprachverstehen. Eine Anleitung zum Gespräch für schwerhörig gewordene Menschen. Neuwied, Berlin: Luchterhand.

Lo, C. Y.; McMahon, C. M.; Looi, V.; Thompson, W. F. (2015): Melodic Contour Training and Its Effect on Speech in Noise, Consonant Discrimination, and Prosody Perception for Cochlear Implant Recipients. In: *Behavioural neurology* 2015, https://doi.org/10.1155/2015/352869

Montano, J. J.; Spitzer, J. B. (2021): Adult Audiologic Rehabilitation. Third Edition. San Diego: Plural Publishing Inc.

Shafiro, V.; Sheft, S.; Kuvadia, S.; Gygi, B. (2015): Environmental sound training in cochlear implant users. In: *Journal of speech, language, and hearing research: JSLHR* 58 (2), S. 509–519. https://doi.org/10.1044/2015_JSLHR-H-14-0312

Wang, W.; Zhou, N.; Xu, L. (2011): Musical pitch and lexical tone perception with cochlear implants. In: *International journal of audiology* 50 (4), S. 270–278. https://doi.org/10.3109/14992027.2010.542490

Zeh, R.; Baumann, U. (2015): Stationäre Rehabilitationsmaßnahmen bei erwachsenen CI-Trägern. Ergebnisse in Abhängigkeit von der Dauer der Taubheit, Nutzungsdauer und Alter. In: *HNO* 63 (8), S. 557–576. https://doi.org/10.1007/s00106-015-0037-2

Exercise Instructions and Materials for Auditory Training

6

In this chapter, you will find exercise material that you can use for the linguistic and nonlinguistic exercise areas mentioned in Chap. 5. The material is merely a basis for therapy and can be expanded as desired by the therapist. The instructions for the exercises do not specify a number of repetitions. When an exercise is finished and the level of difficulty is increased must be decided individually.

▶ The exercise material is also available online at the link: https://link.springer.com/chapter/10.1007/978-3-662-65201-5. The English material with the related DOI is to be included here, instead of the German one

6.1 Exercises of Linguistic Exercise Areas

The following are exercises for the areas of speech sounds, syllables, words, sentences, and texts.

The areas of phoning, as well as listening and understanding in background noise, are excluded at this point, as all other linguistic exercise areas can be embedded in those two areas and considered according to the proposal for increasing difficulty.

Examples for auditory training at the level of everyday communication can be found in the notes of the exercise instructions as well as in Chap. 5.

Supplementary Information The online version contains supplementary material available at https://doi.org/10.1007/978-3-662-72230-5_6.

© The Author(s), under exclusive license to Springer-Verlag GmbH, DE, part of Springer Nature 2025
W. Rötz, B. Bertram, *Cochlear Implantation in Adults*,
https://doi.org/10.1007/978-3-662-72230-5_6

6.1.1 Speech Sounds

6.1.1.1 Differentiating Contrasting Speech Sounds
Presentation of the Exercise Material: Visual
Difficulty level: 1

Instructions: The patient sees two letters or letter combinations that correspond to two contrasting speech sounds. At the beginning, the letters are pronounced as a speech sound once. Then they either hear both speech sounds one after the other or one of the speech sounds twice. The patient decides whether the heard speech sounds are the same or different. The procedure can be repeated several times for the same pair of speech sounds.

Notes: The speech sounds could also be displayed in phonetic script; however, this is not familiar to most patients and can therefore be overwhelming.

It may be necessary to display the choice "same/different" in writing to make the exercise instructions understandable for the patient.

If a pair of speech sounds is used several times in succession, the choice between the same and different is made randomly. Therefore, the same speech sound or both speech sounds can be mentioned twice in a row multiple times. This reduces the probability of guessing.

Material recommendation: See material 01

Presentation of the Exercise Material: Acoustical
Difficulty level: 2

Instructions: The patient hears two acoustically contrasting or two identical speech sounds. The patient decides whether the speech sounds heard are the same or different.

Notes: It may be necessary to present the choice "same/different" in writing to make the exercise instructions understandable for the patient.

Material recommendation: See material 01

6.1.1.2 Differentiating Similar Speech Sounds
Presentation of the Exercise Material: Visual
Difficulty level: 2

Instructions: The patient sees two letters or combinations of letters that correspond to two acoustically similar speech sounds. At the beginning, the letters are pronounced as a speech sound once. Then they hear either both speech sounds one after the other or one of the speech sounds twice. The patient decides whether the speech sounds heard are the same or different. The procedure can be repeated multiple times for the same pair of speech sounds.

Notes: The speech sounds could also be represented in phonetic script, but most patients are not familiar with this, and it could therefore be overwhelming.

It may be necessary to present the choice "same/different" in writing to make the exercise instructions understandable for the patient.

If a pair of speech sounds is used multiple times in a row, the choice between "same and different" is at random. This reduces the probability of guessing.
Material recommendation: See material 01

Presentation of the Exercise Material: Acoustical
Difficulty level: 3
Instructions: The patient hears two acoustically similar or two identical speech sounds. The patient decides whether the speech sounds heard are the same or different.
Notes: It may be necessary to present the choice "same/different" in writing to make the exercise instructions understandable for the patient.
Material recommendation: See material 01

6.1.1.3 Identifying Contrasting Speech Sounds
Presentation of the Exercise Material: Visual
Difficulty level: 1
Instructions: The patient sees three letters or combinations of letters that correspond to three acoustically contrasting speech sounds. At the beginning, the letters are pronounced as a speech sound once. Then the patient hears one of the speech sounds. He decides which speech sound it was. The procedure can be repeated multiple times for the same trio of speech sounds.
Notes: The speech sounds could also be represented in phonetic script, but this is not familiar to most patients and can therefore be overwhelming.

If a speech sound trio is used several times in a row, the selection of the speech sound is at random. So, the same speech sound can be named several times in a row. This reduces the probability of guessing.
Material recommendation: See material 02

6.1.1.4 Identifying Similar Speech Sounds
Presentation of the Exercise Material: Visual
Difficulty level: 2
Instructions: The patient sees three letters or combinations of letters that correspond to three similar speech sounds. At the beginning, the letters are pronounced as a speech sound once. The patient then hears one of the speech sounds. He decides which speech sound it was. The procedure can be repeated several times for the same speech sound trio.
Notes: The speech sounds could also be represented in phonetic script, but this is not familiar to most patients and can therefore be overwhelming.

If a speech sound trio is used several times in a row, the selection of the speech sound is at random. So, the same speech sound can be named several times in a row. This reduces the probability of guessing.
Material recommendation: See material 02

6.1.1.5 Identifying Mixed Speech Sounds
Presentation of the Exercise Material: Acoustical
Difficulty level: 3

Instructions: The patient hears a speech sound and repeats it.

Notes: Patients often repeat heard speech sounds as letters, which is considered correct.

Material recommendation: See materials 01 and 02

6.1.2 Syllables

6.1.2.1 Recognizing Word Length (One Out of Two)
Presentation of the Exercise Material: Visual
Difficulty level: 1

Instructions: The patient sees two similar words of different lengths and hears one of them. He decides which word it was. The procedure can be repeated several times for the same pair of words.

Notes: The goal is to recognize the word length, not to repeat the word. If the patient describes not being able to understand the word well, this is therefore not a mistake.

If a pair of words is used several times in a row, the selection of the word is at random. So, the same word can be named several times in a row. This reduces the probability of guessing.

Material recommendation: See material 03

6.1.2.2 Recognizing Word Length (One Out of Three)
Presentation of the Exercise Material: Visual
Difficulty level: 2

Instructions: The patient sees three similar words of different lengths and hears one of them. He decides which word it was. The procedure can be repeated multiple times for the same trio of words.

Notes: The goal is to recognize the length of the word, not to repeat the word. If the patient describes not being able to understand the word well, this is therefore not a mistake.

If a trio of words is used several times in a row, the selection of the word is at random. So, the same word can be mentioned several times in a row. This reduces the probability of guessing.

Material recommendation: See material 04

6.1.2.3 Detecting the Number of Syllables in a Word
Presentation of the Exercise Material: Acoustical
Difficulty level: 3

Instructions: The patient hears a word and names the number of perceived syllables.

Notes: The goal is to detect the number of syllables, not to repeat the word.

If he still understands and repeats many of the words, this is an additional achievement and indicates that the difficulty can be increased.

Material recommendation: Various words from materials 07, 08, 09, 10, 11, and 12; dictionary; and any books from which random words are selected.

6.1.2.4 Sinking Syllables
Presentation of the Exercise Material: Visual
Difficulty level: 4

Instructions: Sinking syllables is played like "Battleship." In the coordinate system, syllables are named instead of letters and numbers (e.g., not B3, but BA-SO). The patient sees the coordinate system in front of him all the time and repeats the heard syllable combination.

Hints: It should be agreed in advance whether the syllable of the vertical or horizontal row is named first.

Difficult speech sound combinations for the patient can be entered into the empty template to individualize the exercise.

Material recommendation: See material 05

6.1.3 Words

6.1.3.1 Numbers
Presentation of the Exercise Material: Visual
Difficulty level: 1

Instructions: The patient sees five numbers and hears one of them. They decide which number it was. The procedure can be repeated multiple times for the same numbers.

Hints: If a group of numbers is used several times in a row, the selection of the number is at random. So, the same number can be mentioned several times in a row. This reduces the probability of guessing.

Material recommendation: numbers in the range 1–99

Presentation of the Exercise Material: Acoustical
Difficulty level: 2

Instructions: The patient hears a number and repeats it.
Material recommendation: numbers in the range 0–99

6.1.3.2 Words from a Semantic Group (Nouns)
Presentation of the Exercise Material: Visual
Difficulty level: 1

Instructions: The patient gets told a category. He is shown a selection of five words from this category and hears one of them. He decides which word it was. The procedure can be repeated multiple times for the same words.

Notes: The category can be written down and placed in the patient's field of vision if he is struggling to remember it.

Notes: If the words are represented by images, they all need to be named once at the beginning to ensure that the patient associates the correct words with the pictures.

If a word group is used several times in a row, the word is selected at random. Therefore, the same word can be named several times in a row. This reduces the probability of guessing.

Material recommendation: See material 06, theme-specific books, and individual lists (e.g., oriented towards the patient's hobbies and interests)

Presentation of the Exercise Material: Acoustical
Difficulty level: 2

Instructions: The patient gets told a category. They hear a word from this category and repeat it.

Notes: The category can be written down and placed in the patient's field of vision if he is struggling to remember it.

Material recommendation: See material 06, theme-specific books, and individual lists (e.g., oriented towards the patient's hobbies and interests)

6.1.3.3 Tri- to Four-Syllabic Words Without a Semantic Group (Nouns)

Presentation of the Exercise Material: Visual
Difficulty level: 1

Instructions: The patient gets shown a selection of up to eight words and hears one of them. He decides which word it was. The procedure can be repeated multiple times for the same words.

Notes: If the words are represented by images, they all need to be named once at the beginning to ensure that the patient associates the correct words with the pictures.

If a word group is used several times in a row, the word is selected at random. Therefore, the same word can be named several times in a row. This reduces the probability of guessing.

Material recommendation: See material 07, dictionary, novels/articles, etc., from which individual words without a recognizable semantic connection are displayed

Presentation of the Exercise Material: Acoustical
Difficulty level: 2

Instructions: The patient hears a word and repeats it.

Material recommendation: See material 07, dictionary, novels/articles, etc., from which individual words are read out without any recognizable semantic connection

6.1.3.4 Disyllabic Words Without a Semantic Group (Nouns)
Presentation of the Exercise Material: Visual
Difficulty level: 2

Instructions: The patient gets shown a selection of up to eight words and hears one of them. They decide which word it was. The procedure can be repeated multiple times for the same words.

Notes: If the words are represented by images, they all need to be named once at the beginning to ensure that the patient associates the correct words with the pictures.

If a word group is used several times in a row, the word is selected at random. Therefore, the same word can be named several times in a row. This reduces the probability of guessing.

Material recommendation: See material 08, dictionary, novels/articles, etc., from which individual words are displayed without any recognizable semantic connection

Presentation of the Exercise Material: Acoustical
Difficulty level: 3

Instructions: The patient hears a word and repeats it.

Material recommendation: See material 08, dictionary, novels/articles, etc., from which individual words are read out without any recognizable semantic connection

6.1.3.5 Monosyllabic Words Without a Semantic Group (Nouns)
Presentation of the Exercise Material: Visual
Difficulty level: 3

Instructions: The patient is shown a selection of up to eight words and hears one of them. They decide which word it was. The procedure can be repeated multiple times for the same words.

Notes: If the words are represented by images, they all need to be named once at the beginning to ensure that the patient associates the correct words with the pictures.

If a word group is used several times in a row, the word is selected at random. Therefore, the same word can be named several times in a row. This reduces the probability of guessing.

Material recommendation: See material 09, dictionary, novels/articles, etc., from which individual words are displayed without any recognizable semantic connection

Presentation of the Exercise Material: Acoustical
Difficulty level: 4

Instructions: The patient hears a word and repeats it.

Material recommendation: See material 09, dictionary, novels/articles, etc., from which individual words are read out without any recognizable semantic connection

6.1.3.6 Di- to Four-Syllabic Words Without a Semantic Group (All Types of Words)
Presentation of the Exercise Material: Acoustical
Difficulty level: 3
Instructions: The patient hears a word and repeats it.
Material recommendation: See materials 07, 08, 10, and 11; dictionary; novels/articles; etc., from which individual words are read out without any recognizable semantic connection

6.1.3.7 Monosyllabic Without a Semantic Group (All Word Types)
Presentation of the Exercise Material: Acoustical
Difficulty level: 4
Instructions: The patient hears a word and repeats it.
Material recommendation: See materials 09 and 12; dictionary; novels/articles; etc., from which individual words are read out without any recognizable semantic connection

6.1.3.8 Minimal Pairs and Trios (Disyllabic Words)
Presentation of the Exercise Material: Visual
Difficulty level: 2
Instructions: The patient is shown a minimal pair or minimal trio and hears one of the words. They decide which word it was. The procedure can be repeated multiple times for the same words.
Notes: If a minimal pair or trio is used several times in a row, the word is selected at random. Therefore, the same word can be named several times in a row. This reduces the probability of guessing.
If the exercise is performed with minimal pairs, this increases the probability of a randomly correct assignment compared to the execution with minimal trios.
Material recommendation: See materials 13 and 14

Presentation of the Exercise Material: Acoustical
Difficulty level: 3
Instructions: The patient hears two or three words (a minimal pair or trio) directly one after the other and then repeats all the words at once.
Notes: Both words should be emphasized in the same way.
Material recommendation: See materials 13 and 14

6.1.3.9 Minimal Pairs and Trios (Monosyllabic Words)
Presentation of the Exercise Material: Visual
Difficulty level: 2
Instructions: The patient is shown a minimal pair or trio and hears one of the words. He decides which word it was. The procedure can be repeated multiple times for the same words.

Notes: If a minimal pair or trio is used several times in a row, the word is selected at random. Therefore, the same word can be named several times in a row. This reduces the probability of guessing.

If the exercise is performed with minimal pairs, this increases the probability of a randomly correct assignment compared to the execution with minimal trios.

Material recommendation: See materials 15 and 16

Presentation of the Exercise Material: Acoustical
Difficulty level: 3

Instructions: The patient hears two or three words (a minimal pair or trio) directly one after the other and then repeats all the words at once.

Notes: Both words should be emphasized in the same way.

Material recommendation: See materials 15 and 16

6.1.3.10 Compound Noun
Presentation of the Exercise Material: Mixed Acoustical and Visual
Difficulty level: 1

Instructions: The patient sees a part of a compound noun and hears the entire word. They then repeat the entire word.

Notes: It must be made clear to the patient which part of the word is visualized. A numbered template on which the visual part is labelled 1 or 2 is suitable for this.

Material recommendation: See material 17

6.1.3.11 Words from an Extended Semantic Group with an Umbrella Term
Presentation of the Exercise Material: Acoustical
Difficulty level: 2

Instructions: The patient gets told an umbrella term. The patient hears one of the five words at a time related to the umbrella term and repeats each of them.

Notes: The umbrella term can be written down and placed in the patient's field of vision if he is struggling to remember it.

Material recommendation: See material 18 and cards from the game "TABOO"

6.1.3.12 Words from an Extended Semantic Group Without an Umbrella Term
Presentation of the Exercise Material: Acoustical
Difficulty level: 3

Instructions: The patient hears one of five words at a time related to an umbrella term, which is not given to them in advance, and repeats them one after another. The patient must remember the five words and try to guess the described umbrella term based on them.

Material recommendation: See material 18 and cards from the game "TABOO"

6.1.3.13 Names
Presentation of the Exercise Material: Acoustical
Difficulty level: 3
   Instructions: The patient hears a name and repeats it.
   Material recommendation: See material 19

6.1.3.14 Hidden Object Pictures
Presentation of the Exercise Material: Acoustical
Difficulty level: 3
   Instructions: The patient hears one of three words at a time and repeats them one after another. The words describe an object or a person in a hidden object picture. The patient has to memorize the words and then look for the corresponding object or person in the picture.
   Material recommendation: Detailed pictures for adults or children (in books or via Google search)

6.1.3.15 Foreign Words—Rare Words
Presentation of the Exercise Material: Acoustical
Difficulty level: 4
   Instructions: The patient hears a word and repeats it.
   Material recommendation: See material 20, foreign word dictionary, and specialist books or dictionaries on a specific topic (e.g., medical books)

6.1.3.16 Speech Sound Twisters
Presentation of the Exercise Material: Acoustical
Difficulty level: 4
   Instructions: The patient hears a "twisted" word and repeats it as incorrectly as they were pronounced. Then they try to name the original word by swapping the previously twisted speech sounds.
   Notes: The exercise should be carried out entirely acoustically. The patient should also try to "swap back" without a written image to create an additional cognitive demand.
   Material recommendation: See material 21 and dictionary

6.1.4 Phrases

6.1.4.1 Gap Phrases from a Semantic Group
Presentation of the Exercise Material: Mixed Acoustical and Visual
Difficulty level: 1
   Instructions: The patient gets told a category. They see a gapped phrase of this category and hear the complete phrase. They repeat the missing word or the complete phrase.
   Notes: The category can be written down and placed in the patient's field of vision if they are struggling to remember it.

Material recommendation: See material 22

6.1.4.2 Gap Phrases Without a Semantic Group
Presentation of the Exercise Material: Mixed Acoustical and Visual
Difficulty level: 2
Instructions: The patient sees a gapped phrase and hears the complete phrase. They repeat the missing word or the complete phrase.
Material recommendation: See material 23

6.1.4.3 Phrases in the Semantic Group
Presentation of the Exercise Material: Acoustical
Difficulty level: 2
Instructions: The patient gets told a category. The patient hears a phrase of this category and repeats it.
Notes: The category can be written down and placed in the patient's field of vision if they are struggling to remember it.
Material recommendation: See material 24

6.1.4.4 Phrases from an Extended Semantic Group
Presentation of the Exercise Material: Acoustical
Difficulty level: 2
Instructions: The patient gets told a category. The patient hears a phrase from this category and repeats it.
Notes: The category can be written down and placed in the patient's field of vision if they are struggling to remember it.
Material recommendation: See material 25, ingredient lists from baking and cooking books, and material lists from craft books

6.1.4.5 Idioms
Presentation of the Exercise Material: Acoustical
Difficulty level: 2
Instructions: The patient hears an idiom and repeats it.
Notes: This exercise only has a difficulty level of two for patients for whom idioms are part of the automated speech. Otherwise, the difficulty level increases.
Material recommendation: See material 26

6.1.4.6 Phrases Without a Semantic Group
Presentation of the Exercise Material: Acoustical
Difficulty level: 3
Instructions: The patient hears a phrase and repeats it.
Material recommendation: See material 27

6.1.4.7 Paraphrases Without an Umbrella Term
Presentation of the Exercise Material: Acoustical
Difficulty level: 4

Instructions: The patient hears the paraphrase of a word and repeats it. Then, they try to find out the sought word.

Notes: In the subsequent solution finding, the therapist can support the patient through targeted questions and descriptions. The patient continues to look away. In this way, the exercise is elevated to a communicative level.

Material recommendation: See material 28 and paraphrases of various sweets or manufacturers of sweets via the Google search for "candy quiz"

6.1.5 Sentences

6.1.5.1 Short Sentences
Presentation of the Exercise Material: Visual
Difficulty level: 1

Instructions: The patient sees a selection of three sentences and hears one of them. He decides which sentence it was. The procedure can be repeated multiple times for the same sentences.

Notes: If a group of sentences is used several times in a row, the sentence is selected at random. Therefore, the same sentence can be repeated several times in a row. This reduces the probability of guessing.

Material recommendation: See material 29

Presentation of the Exercise Material: Acoustical
Difficulty level: 2

Instructions: The patient hears a sentence and repeats it.
Material recommendation: See material 29

6.1.5.2 Gap Sentences from a Semantic Group
Presentation of the Exercise Material: Mixed Acoustical and Visual
Difficulty level: 1

Instructions: The patient gets told a category. They see a gapped sentence of this category and hear the complete sentence. The patient repeats the missing word or the complete sentence.

Notes: The category can be written down and placed in the patient's field of vision if they are struggling to remember it.

Material recommendation: See material 30

6.1.5.3 Sentences from a Semantic Group
Presentation of the Exercise Material: Acoustical
Difficulty level: 2

Instructions: The patient gets told a category. The patient hears a sentence of this category and repeats it.

Notes: The category can be written down and placed in the patient's field of vision if they are struggling to remember it.
Material recommendation: See material 31

6.1.5.4 Proverbs
Presentation of the Exercise Material: Acoustical
Difficulty level: 2
Instructions: The patient hears a proverb and repeats it.
Notes: This exercise only has a difficulty level 2 for patients for whom proverbs are part of their automated language. Otherwise, the difficulty level increases.
Material recommendation: See material 32 and correct proverbs from material 35

6.1.5.5 Gap Sentences Without a Semantic Group
Presentation of the Exercise Material: Mixed Acoustical and Visual
Difficulty level: 2
Instructions: The patient sees a sentence with a gap and hears the complete sentence. He repeats the missing word or the complete sentence.
Material recommendation: See material 33

6.1.5.6 Paraphrases with an Umbrella Term
Presentation of the Exercise Material: Acoustical
Difficulty level: 2
Instructions: The patient gets told an umbrella term. The patient hears a paraphrase related to the umbrella term and repeats it.
Notes: The umbrella term can be written down and placed in the patient's field of vision if they are struggling to remember it.
Material recommendation: See material 34 and cards from the game "20 Questions"

6.1.5.7 Proverbs with Similar Words
Presentation of the Exercise Material: Acoustical
Difficulty level: 3
Instructions: The patient hears a correct or slightly altered, incorrect proverb and repeats it as incorrectly or correctly as it was spoken.
Notes: This exercise only has difficulty level 3 for patients for whom proverbs are part of automated speech. Otherwise, the difficulty level may decrease, as the patient is not able to mentally complete the proverb before it is completely spoken. This makes incorrect words more likely to be heard.
Material recommendation: See material 35

6.1.5.8 Simple Nonsense Sentences
Presentation of the Exercise Material: Acoustical
Difficulty level: 3
Instructions: The patient hears a sentence and repeats it.
Material recommendation: See material 36

6.1.5.9 Difficult Nonsense Sentences
Presentation of the Exercise Material: Acoustical
Difficulty level: 4
    Instructions: The patient hears a sentence and repeats it.
    Material recommendation: See material 37

6.1.5.10 Hidden Object Pictures
Presentation of the Exercise Material: Acoustical
Difficulty level: 4
    Instructions: The patient hears one of three sentences at a time and repeats them one after another. The sentences describe an object or a person in a hidden object picture. The patient has to memorize the sentences and then look for the corresponding object or person in the picture.
    Material recommendation: hidden object pictures for adults or children (in books or via Google Search)

6.1.5.11 Sentences in the Extended Semantic Group Without an Umbrella Term
Presentation of the Exercise Material: Acoustical
Difficulty level: 4
    Instructions: The patient hears one sentence at a time related to an umbrella term, which is not given to them in advance, and repeats them one after another. The patient must remember the sentences and try to guess the described umbrella term based on them.
    Material recommendation: See material 34 and cards from the game "20 Questions"

6.1.5.12 Complex Sentences
Presentation of the Exercise Material: Acoustical
Difficulty level: 4
    Instructions: The patient hears a sentence and repeats it.
    Material recommendation: See material 38, novels/articles, etc., from which individual longer or content-wise complex sentences without recognizable semantic context are read aloud; and various quiz games at the sentence level with three to four answer options each

6.1.5.13 Quotes
Presentation of the Exercise Material: Acoustical
Difficulty level: 4
    Instructions: The patient hears a quote and repeats it.
    Material recommendation: See material 39

6.1.6 Texts

6.1.6.1 Reading Along
Presentation of the Exercise Material: Mixed Acoustical and Visual
Difficulty level: 1

Instructions: The therapist reads out a text that the patient also has in front of them. The patient follows the text only with their eyes, without reading aloud. The therapist stops the reading at any point, and the patient repeats the last word read. Then, the reading continues.

Notes: Initially, sections or paragraphs that will be read can also be determined together. After each section or paragraph, the patient gives feedback on whether they were able to follow the text up to this point.

Material recommendation: Various books, magazines, newspapers, etc.

6.1.6.2 Phrase by Phrase
Presentation of the Exercise Material: Acoustical
Difficulty level: 2

Instructions: The therapist reads out a short text phrase by phrase. The patient repeats each one and tries to grasp the content of the text in the process.

Notes: If the patient reports back afterwards not having been able to follow the content of the text, the text can be read again completely in one piece.

Material recommendation: Short stories and short articles

Presentation of the Exercise Material: Acoustical
Difficulty level: 3

Instructions: The therapist reads out a poem verse by verse, with the patient repeating the individual verses.

Notes: Poems should be chosen that do not leave too much room for interpretation in their content or are not too complex in content.

Material recommendation: Volumes of poetry and song lyrics

6.1.6.3 Text Comprehension
Presentation of the Exercise Material: Acoustical
Difficulty level: 3–4

Instructions: A text is read out to the patient. Subsequently, he summarizes the content of the text or answers questions about the text.

Notes: If the text is very long, it can also be approached section by section or paragraph by paragraph.

The difficulty level of the exercise is varied through the content and linguistic complexity of the text.

Material recommendation: Short stories and newspaper articles

6.2 Exercises for Nonlinguistic Exercise Areas

The following exercises are suitable for the areas of noise, tone, melody and music, and voice.

The area of spatial hearing is excluded at this point, as this is best combined with other exercise areas in practice. Concrete suggestions for integrating spatial hearing into therapy can be found in Chap. 5.

6.2.1 Noises

6.2.1.1 Differentiating Contrasting Noises
Presentation of the Exercise Material: Acoustical
Difficulty level: 1

Instructions: The patient hears two acoustically contrasting noises. The patient decides whether the heard noises are the same or different.

Notes: It may be necessary to present the choice "same/different" in writing to make the exercise instructions understandable for the patient.

If the therapist makes the noises themselves, the patient should close their eyes, if possible, as this may require larger physical movements.

Contrasts can be achieved through different noise lengths (e.g., rubbing hands vs. clapping) and frequency ranges (e.g., knocking vs. whistling).

Material recommendation: CDs with recorded noises, percussion instruments, noise memory game, and self-produced noises (e.g., clapping, snapping, whistling, rubbing hands, scratching, stomping, knocking, clearing throat, rustling paper...)

6.2.1.2 Differentiating Similar Noises
Presentation of the Exercise Material: Acoustical
Difficulty level: 2

Instructions: The patient hears two acoustically similar noises. The patient decides whether the heard noises are the same or different.

Notes: It may be necessary to present the choice "same/different" in writing to make the exercise instructions understandable for the patient.

If the therapist makes the noises themselves, the patient should close their eyes, if possible, as this may require larger physical movements. Contrasts can be achieved through different noise lengths (e.g., rubbing hands vs. clapping) and frequency ranges (e.g., knocking vs. whistling).

Material recommendation: CDs with recorded noises, percussion instruments, noise memory game, and self-produced noises (e.g., clapping, snapping, whistling, rubbing hands, scratching, stomping, knocking, clearing throat, rustling paper...)

6.2.1.3 Identifying Everyday Noises
Presentation of the Exercise Material: Visual
Difficulty level: 3

Instructions: The patient sees a selection of ten images of everyday noises and hears one of them. They decide which noise it was.

Notes: In conversation, properties of the noises can be discussed in advance, or, as an assisting technique, after listening.

Material recommendation: CDs with recorded everyday noises

6.2.1.4 Noise Memory Game
Presentation of the Exercise Material: Acoustical
Difficulty level: 3–4

Instructions: The noise memory game is played according to the rules of a normal memory game. The patient and the therapist alternately choose two noise cans, listen to them in comparison, and decide whether they are the same or different.

Notes: The aim is not for the patient to find out what the noise cans contain. Given the variety of sounds, this is mostly not possible even with normal hearing.

When comparing noises, properties of the noise should be discussed that result from the sound of the noise (loud or quiet, high or low, hard or soft, one part or several, large or small, etc.). This provides additional clues for the CI fitting. The more pairs the memory game contains, the higher the difficulty level, as the patient has to remember more items.

Material recommendation: Noise memory game (opaque containers filled with everyday objects and materials such as legumes, paper clips, coins, nuts, dried flowers/leaves, pins, stones, etc.)

6.2.2 Tones

6.2.2.1 Differentiating Contrasting Tones (>3 Half Steps)
Presentation of the Exercise Material: Acoustical
Difficulty level: 2

Instructions: The patient hears two contrasting or two same tones. The patient decides whether both are the same or different.

Notes: It may be necessary to present the choice "same/different" in writing to make the exercise instructions understandable for the patient.

The exercise can be performed in different frequency ranges and on different instruments.

Material recommendation: Instruments and instrument app (e.g., piano)

6.2.2.2 Differentiating Similar Tones (<3 Half Steps)
Presentation of the Exercise Material: Acoustical
Difficulty level: 3

Instructions: The patient hears two similar or two same tones. The patient decides whether both are the same or different.

Notes: It may be necessary to present the choice "same/different" in writing to make the exercise instructions understandable for the patient.

The exercise can be performed in different frequency ranges and on various instruments.

Material recommendation: Instruments and instrument app (e.g., piano)

6.2.2.3 Identifying Contrasting Tones (>3 Half Steps)
Presentation of the Exercise Material: Acoustical
Difficulty level: 3

Instructions: The patient hears two opposite tones. The patient decides which tone was the higher or lower one.

Notes: The exercise can be performed in different frequency ranges and on various instruments.

Material recommendation: Instruments and instrument app (e.g., piano)

6.2.2.4 Identifying Similar Tones (<3 Half Steps)
Presentation of the Exercise Material: Acoustical
Difficulty level: 3

Instructions: The patient hears two similar tones. The patient decides which tone was the higher or lower one.

Notes: The exercise can be performed in different frequency ranges and on various instruments.

Material recommendation: Instruments and instrument app (e.g., piano)

6.2.2.5 Identifying Tones
Presentation of the Exercise Material: Acoustical
Difficulty level: 4

Instructions: The patient hears three tones, at least two of which are different. The patient decides in which order they were played.

Notes: It can be differentiated into high, medium, and low tones. This results in various combinations like "high-high-low," "low-medium-high," "low-high-medium," etc.

Material recommendation: Instruments and instrument app (e.g., piano)

6.2.3 Melody and Music

6.2.3.1 Differentiating Melodies
Presentation of the Exercise Material: Acoustical
Difficulty level: 2

Instructions: The patient hears two melodies and decides whether both are the same or different.

Notes: It does not have to be a well-known melody. Any sequence of tones can be used. The exercise can be performed in different frequency ranges and on various instruments.

It may be necessary to present the choice "same/different" in writing to make the exercise instructions understandable for the patient.

Material recommendation: Instruments and instrument app (e.g., piano)

6.2.3.2 Identifying Voices
Presentation of Exercise Material: Acoustical
Difficulty level: 3

Instructions: The patient listens to a song with vocals and decides whether it is sung by a man or a woman.

Notes: To increase the difficulty, songs with multiple singers can also be used.

Material recommendation: Playback device including speakers or the ability to directly connect the patient's additional technical accessories, CDs, access to music streaming services, and YouTube

6.2.3.3 Identifying Instruments
Presentation of Exercise Material: Acoustical
Difficulty level: 3

Instructions: The patient listens to a song in sections. After each section, the song is paused, and the patient decides which instrument or if a voice has been added.

Notes: This exercise requires some preparation, as the therapist must divide the songs in advance.

It is recommended to start with songs that contain only a few instruments and voices and to increase the difficulty over an increasing number of instruments and voices from song to song.

Material recommendation: Playback device including speakers or the ability to directly connect the patient's additional technical accessories, CDs, access to music streaming services, and YouTube

6.2.3.4 Identifying Melodies
Presentation of Exercise Material: Acoustical
Difficulty level: 3

Instructions: The patient listens to a melody of a known song played with a single instrument (e.g., children's songs) and decides which one it is.

Notes: The melody can either be played live by the therapist or played from an audio source (e.g., from a CD or online).

Favorite bands or titles can be asked beforehand to ensure that the songs are known to the patient.

Material recommendation: Playback device including speakers or the ability to directly connect the patient's additional technical accessories, CDs, access to music streaming services, and YouTube

6.2.3.5 Identifying Language
Presentation of Exercise Material: Visual
Difficulty level: 3

Instructions: The patient listens to a song and is given four possible languages to choose from. The patient decides in which of the languages the song was sung.

Notes: This exercise can also be carried out without a selection. However, due to the large number of languages, this is very demanding. Identifying the language can be well combined with the exercises "Identifying Instruments" and "Identifying Voices."

Material recommendation: Playback device including speakers or the ability to directly connect the patient's additional technical accessories, CDs, access to music streaming services, and YouTube

6.2.3.6 Identifying Songs
Presentation of the Exercise Material: Acoustical
Difficulty level: 4

Instructions: The patient listens to the recording of a known song and decides which song it is.

Notes: Favorite bands or titles can be asked beforehand to ensure that the songs are known to the patient.

Material recommendation: Playback device including speakers or the ability to directly connect the patient's additional technical accessories, CDs, access to music streaming services, and YouTube

6.2.3.7 Identifying Texts
Presentation of the Exercise Material: Acoustical
Difficulty level: 4

Instructions: The patient listens to the recording of a song in their native language and describes what the song is about or names text passages that they can understand.

Notes: For this exercise, the played songs should be largely unknown.

Material recommendation: Playback device including speakers or the ability to directly connect the patient's additional technical accessories, CDs, access to music streaming services, and YouTube

6.2.4 Voices

6.2.4.1 Differentiating Voices
Presentation of the Exercise Material: Acoustical
Difficulty level: 2

Instructions: The patient listens to two speakers and decides whether they are the same or different.

Notes: If the same speaker is played twice, it can either be the same recording or two different recordings of a speaker.

It may be necessary to present the choice "same/different" in writing to make the exercise instructions understandable for the patient.

6.2 Exercises for Nonlinguistic Exercise Areas

Material recommendation: Playback device including speakers or the ability to directly connect the patient's additional technical accessories, CDs, access to movie and TV streaming services or media libraries, and YouTube

6.2.4.2 Identifying Voices (Male/Female)
Presentation of the Exercise Material: Acoustical
Difficulty level: 3

Instructions: The patient listens to a speaker and decides whether it is a man or a woman.

Material recommendation: Playback device including speakers or the ability to directly connect the patient's additional technical accessories, CDs, access to movie and TV streaming services or media libraries, and YouTube

6.2.4.3 Identifying Voices (Adult/Child)
Presentation of the Exercise Material: Acoustical
Difficulty level: 3

Instructions: The patient listens to a speaker and decides whether it is an adult or a child.

Material recommendation: Playback device including speakers or the ability to directly connect the patient's additional technical accessories, CDs, access to movie and TV streaming services or media libraries, and YouTube

6.2.4.4 Identifying Known Voices
Presentation of the Exercise Material: Visually
Difficulty level: 3

Instructions: The patient listens to a speaker and chooses from a selection of 3 speakers the correct one.

Notes: Suitable voices are of politicians, newsreaders, presenters, actors, or other public figures. The patient can be asked beforehand which movies they know well or which television channels or television shows they watch more frequently, to ensure that the persons are known.

Material recommendation: Playback device including speakers or the ability to directly connect the patient's additional technical accessories, CDs, access to movie and TV streaming services or media libraries, and YouTube

Presentation of the Exercise Material: Acoustical
Difficulty level: 4

Instructions: The patient listens to a speaker and decides which person it is.

Notes: Suitable voices are of politicians, newsreaders, presenters, actors, or other public figures. The patient can be asked beforehand which movies he knows well or which television channels or television shows he watches more frequently, to ensure that the persons are known.

Material recommendation: Playback device including speakers or the ability to directly connect the patient's additional technical accessories, CDs, access to movie and TV streaming services or media libraries, and YouTube

Glossary

Advanced Bionics (AB) CI manufacturer
Aided threshold Hearing threshold with device support, measured in the sound field
Auditory Brainstem Implant (ABI) An implant that attaches to the brainstem to make acoustic signals audible again
Bilateral On both sides
Bimodal Different device support for each ear
Binaural In both ears
C-Level Here: Threshold of comfortable loudness in CI fitting
Coarticulation Articulatory adjustment of a sound to the surrounding sounds during speech
Cochlear® CI manufacturer
CROS system Hearing aid with devices behind the ears (similar to behind-the-ear hearing aids), where the device behind the deaf ear transmits incoming signals with a time delay to the device on the well-hearing side
Deaf community Community of the deaf
Dichotic hearing Simultaneous hearing of two different acoustic signals in both ears
Directional characteristic Here: Setting of direction and sensitivity, how incoming sounds are processed by the processor microphones of the CI
Earmold Custom-fitted ear piece
Extracochlear Outside the cochlea
Insertion Here: Of the electrode carrier into the cochlea
Intracochlear Inside the cochlea
Lateral At the side
Lip-seeing Here: Lipreading to supplement auditory information
Live-Voice Here: Conducting exercises with live spoken language
Masking Unilateral, artificially induced hearing loss or deafness, e.g., through noise in hearing tests or in auditory training
MED-EL CI manufacturer
Monaural In one ear
Nurotron® CI manufacturer
Oticon Medical (OM) CI manufacturer

Percutaneous Through an intentionally opened skin site
Postlingual After the completion of language acquisition
Postoperative After the operation
Prelingual Before the completion of language acquisition
Reimplantation Replacement of an implant (e.g., due to a defect)
Remote CI fitting CI fitting from a distance
Single-Sided Deafness (SSD) Unilateral deafness with normal hearing on the opposite side
Speech processor Here: External part of the CI system
Speech coding strategy Strategies by which recorded speech is processed
T-Level Here: Hearing threshold in CI fitting
Tinnitus suppression Reducing the perception of tinnitus
Transcutaneous Through the skin while the skin remains intact
Upgrade Here: Provision with a speech processor of a newer generation

Index

A
ABI (Auditory brainstem implant), 31
Acceptance, 66
ACIR (Working Group for Cochlear Implant Rehabilitation), 6, 31
Adapting hearing systems in bilateral/bimodal supply, 90
Additional technical accessories, 56
    alarm devices, 52, 53
    CI manufacturer, 56
    everyday use, 89
    telephones, 53, 54
Aided threshold, 71
Alarm devices, 52–53
Assisting techniques, auditory training, 100–106
    level 1, 100, 101
    level 2, 101, 105
    level 3, 105, 106
    transcript, 106, 108
Audio source, instructions for use, 48
Auditory brainstem implant (ABI), 31
Auditory deconditioning, 38
Auditory therapy
    educational offerings, 43
Audiotory training
    assisting techniques, 100, 106
    exercise sequence, 82
    foreign language, 50, 51
    goal, auditory training, 46
    interpreters, 54
    non-linguistic and linguistic exercise areas, 79
    prerequisite, auditory training, 45
    report, 46
    secure communication, 99
    starting level, 72
    terminoligies, 41
    video chat, 49, 50

B
Basic rules of exercise execution, 83–87
    beginning of therapy, 84
    interdisciplinary exchange with CI technicians, 87
    recognizing patient fatigue, 87
    temporary masking of the opposite ear, 84, 85
    understanding without lip-seeing, 86
    volume setting, 85, 86
Beginning of therapy, 84
Behind-the-ear processor, 14–16
Bilateral, 5, 30, 36
Bimodal, 36
Binaural, 30
Brain plasticity, 26, 44

C
Cable transmission, 54
Causes, 6
Central, 31
Coarticulation, 44, 87

Cochlear implant (CI)
    CI manufacturer, 10, 11, 56
        additional technical
            accessories, 56
        contact details, 11
    CI technician, 63
        fitting options, 64
    implantation, 63
    Keidel, Wolf-Dieter, 2
    single channel implant, 3
    supply
        bilateral, 5, 30, 36
        bimodal, 36
        complications, 37
        goal, implantation, 32
        guideline, 31
        indication, 29
        occupational reintegration, 33
        single-sided-deafness, 5, 31
        unilateral, 36
    Zöllner, Frank, 2
Cocktail party effect, 26
Cognitive performance, in communication, 81
Complications, 37
Consequences, 28, 66
Contact details, 11
Current sound processors, 17

D
Deaf community, 4, 38
Diagnostics
    aided threshold, 71
    monosyllabic test, 71
    multisyllabic test, 71
    speech tracking, 70
    vowel and consonant
        identification, 69
Djourno, André, 2

E
EAS (electro-acoustic stimulation), 5, 30
Education offers, 43
Electro-acoustic stimulation (EAS), 5, 30
Electrode array, 10
Electrodes, CI, 10
Erber, Norman P., hearing development, 77
Exchange, interdisciplinary, 46
Everyday communication, 88–90
Everyday life, 93
Everyday use, 89
Exchange, 46

Exercise areas
    everyday communication, 88, 90
    hearing and understanding
        in noise, 90, 91
    melody and music, 96
    noises, 94, 95
    phone calls, 91, 94
    tones, 95
    spatial hearing, 97, 98
    speech sounds, 87
    weighting, contentual, 80
        cognitive performance,
            in communication, 81
        linguistic parameters, 80
        presentation of exercise
            material, 81, 83
    words, phrases, sentences and texts, 88
    voices, 96
Exercise instructions
    melody and music, 132, 134
    noises, 130, 131
    phrases, 124, 126
    sentences, 126, 128
    speech sounds, 116, 118
    syllables, 118, 119
    texts, 129
    tones, 131, 132
    voices, 134, 135
    words, 119, 124
Exercise sequence, 82
Eyriès, Charles, 2

F
Fitting, 18, 64
Foreign language, 50–51
Freiburg monosyllabic test, 71
Freiburg number test, 71
Function of hearing, 25–27
Functions of human HEARING ability, 27

G
Goal, 32, 46
Guideline, 31

H
Hearing
    binaural, 30
    function of hearing, 25, 27
    sensory performance, 25
    and understanding in noise, 90–91

Hearing disorders
    causes, 6
    central, 31
    consequences, in age, 29
    acceptance, psychosocial consequences, 66
    function of human hearing ability, consequences, 27
    pronunciation, 65
House, William, single channel implant, 3

I
ICF (International Clasification of Functioning, Disability and Health), 42, 65, 72, 74
Illiteracy, 68
Implant
    electrodes, 10
    electrode array, 10
    implantable part, 9, 10
    properties, 12, 13
    receiver coil, 9
    stimulator, 9
Implantable part, 9–10
Implantation, 63
Independent training at home, 98–99
Indication, 29
Inductive transmission, 9
Interdisciplinary Exchange with CI Technicians, 87
International Classification of Functioning, Disability and Health (ICF), 42, 65, 72–74
Interpreters, 50

K
Keidel, Wolf-Dieter, 2
Kinem (mouth shape), 86

L
Level 1, 100–101
Level 2, 101–105
Level 3, 105–106
Levels of hearing development, 77
Linguistic parameters, 80
Lip-reading, 86
Lip-seeing, 86

M
Making phone calls, 93
    everyday life, 93
    with the CI, alternatives, 93

Masking, 85
Melody and music, 96, 132–134
Menière's disease, 7
Monosyllabic test, 71
Mouth shape (kinem), 86
Multisyllabic test, 71

N
Noises, exercise area, 94, 95
Noises, exercises, 130, 131
Non-linguistic and linguistic exercise areas, 79

O
Obliteration, 3, 7, 12, 29
Occupational reintegration, 33
Online therapies, 49
Ossification, 3, 7, 12
Outpatient *vs.* inpatient rehabilitation, 51–52

P
Patient mentors, 37
Phone calls, 91–94
Phrases, 88, 124–126
Plasticity of brain, 26, 44
Possibilities, 98
Possibilities of technical adjustments, 109
Power supply, sound processor, 8
Prerequisite, 45, 49
Presentation of exercise material, 81–83
Prognosis, hearing success, 68
Pronunciation, 65
Properties, 12–13

R
Receiver coil, 9
Recognizing patient fatigue, 87
Reimplantation, 37

S
Secure communication, 99
Self-help groups, 44
Sensory performance, 25
Sentences, 88, 126–128
Setting options, 64
Sign language, 68
Single channel implant, 3

Single-sided-deafness (SSD), 5, 31
   consequences, 66
   masking, 85
   online therapy, 49
   training via direct connection, 48
Single-unit processors, making phone calls, 16–17, 93
Sound processor, 8
   behind-the-ear processor, 14, 16
   current sound processors, 17
   fitting, 18, 64
   possibilities of technical adjustments, 109
   single-unit processor, 16, 17
   wearing time, 98
Spatial hearing, exercise area, 97–98
Special features, 50
Speech sounds, exercise area, 87, 116–118
Speech-tracking, 70
SSD (Single-sided-deafness), 5, 31
Starting level, 72
Stimulator, 9
Syllables, 118–119

T
Telemetry, 6
Telephones, 53–54
Temporary masking of opposite ear, 84–85
Terminologies, 41
Texts, 88, 129
Therapy via video chat
   prerequisite, 49
   special features, 50
Tones, exercise area, 95, 131–132
Totally implantable cochlear implant (TICI), 5

Training via a direct connection, 48
Transcript, 106–108
Transmission paths, 54–56
   wireless transmission, 54, 56
   cable transmission, 54
Transmitter coil, 9
   inductive transmission, 9

U
Understanding without lip-seeing, 86
Unilateral, 36
Urban, Jack, single channel implant, 3
Useful sound, 90

V
Video chat, 49–50
Voices, 96, 134–135
Volta, Alessandro, 1
Volume setting, 85–86
Vowel and consonant identification, 69

W
Wearing time, 98
Weighting, 80
William House and Jack Urban, 3
Wireless transmission, 54–56
Words, 88, 119–124
Working Group for Cochlear Implant Rehabilitation (ACIR), 6, 31

Z
Zöllner, Frank, 2

MIX
Papier aus verantwortungsvollen Quellen
Paper from responsible sources
FSC® C105338

If you have any concerns about our products,
you can contact us on
ProductSafety@springernature.com

In case Publisher is established outside the EU,
the EU authorized representative is:
**Springer Nature Customer Service Center GmbH
Europaplatz 3, 69115 Heidelberg, Germany**

Printed by Libri Plureos GmbH
in Hamburg, Germany